RESEARCH AND PERSPECTIVES IN LONGEVITY

Springer

Berlin
Heidelberg
New York
Hong Kong
London
Milan
Paris
Tokyo

C. E. Finch J.-M. Robine Y. Christen (Eds.)

Brain and Longevity

With 32 Figures and 20 Tables

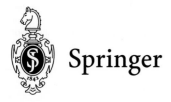

Springer

Finch, Caleb E.
Ethel Percy Aandrus Gerontology Center
Division of Neurogerontology
University Park MC-0191
3715 Mc Clintok
Los Angeles, CA 90089-0191
USA

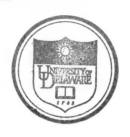

Robine, Jean-Marie
INSERM
Equipe Demographie et Sante
Centre Val d'aurelle
Parc Euromedecine
34298 Montpellier cedex
France
Email: robine@valdorel.fnclcc.fr

Christen, Yves, Ph.D.
Fondation IPSEN
Pour la Recherche Thérapeutique
24, rue Erlanger
75781 Paris Cedex 16
France
Email: yves.christen@beaufour-ipsen.com

ISBN 3-540-43958-7   Springer-Verlag Berlin Heidelberg New York

Library of Congress-Cataloging-in-Publication-Data

Brain and longevity / C.E. Finch, J.-M. Robin, Y. Christen (eds.). p. cm. – (Research and perspectives in longevity)
  Includes bibliographical references and index.
  ISBN 3540439587 (alk. paper)
1. Longevity. 2. Brain-Aging. 3. Cognition. 4. Evolution. 5. Brain-Evolution. I. Finch, Caleb Ellicott. II. Robine, Jean-Marie. III. Christen, Yves. IV. Series.

Springer-Verlag a member of BertelsmannSpringer
Science + Business Media GmbH
http://www.springer.de

© Springer-Verlag Berlin Heidelberg 2003
Printed in Germany

Production: PRO EDIT GmbH, 69126 Heidelberg, Germany
Cover design: design & production, 69121 Heidelberg, Germany
Printed on acid-free paper   SPIN: 10884765   27/3135Re – 5 4 3 2 1 0

Preface

The Fondation IPSEN has been organizing international symposiums on Alzheimer's disease and neurosciences for more than 10 years, and on longevity since 5 years ago. It stands to reason that these two major themes should be associated in the same symposium. Thus, the Fondation IPSEN chose to devote one of its "Colloque Médecine et Recherche" to "Brain and longevity". The symposium was held in Paris on October 8, 2001, and surprisingly it was the first one on this theme. Yet, reading the articles of these proceedings, one discerns the essential relationship between the brain and longevity. They are not only two themes joined together for convenience in a symposium intending to gather biologists and demographers, but two interpenetrating domains. Several times, it clearly appeared that researchers from both sides were bringing together pieces of the same puzzle.

While summarizing the "Brain and Longevity" symposium in the newsletter *Alzheimer Actualités* dated January–February 2002, Jennifer Altman reminds us that, "our brains are three to four times bigger than those of our cousins the great apes", and that "we live about twice as long". It is all a matter of questions! Is there a correlation between brain size and longevity? Have these parameters evolved in parallel? What biologic mechanism do they rest on? What influence may the brain have on longevity and what are its mechanisms? And conversely, what may be the influence of longevity on the brain and its functioning?

The fourth symposium of the Fondation IPSEN devoted to longevity tried to answer these questions, both at the level of the species and at the level of contemporary human populations. It followed on from the first symposium which was devoted to the limits of human longevity (1996), and the other two on the paradoxes of longevity (1998) and sexuality, gender, reproduction and parenthood (1999). Each theme adopted by the Fondation IPSEN has allowed the organization of a multidisciplinary team, including anthropologists, biologists, demographers, epidemiologists, geneticists, physicians, nutritionists, and sociologists ... for the best scientific debate.

From the Blanding turtle to humans through to chimpanzees, experience appears to be a fundamental element for a long survival. Among the factors contributing to the increase of both brain size and longevity are: the prematurity of young humans; the long period of dependency and long period of experience and learning linked to the mode of nutrition; and the appearance of the E3 allele on the gene of apolipoprotein E between 600,000 and 175,000 years ago, allowing the oldest post-reproductive humans to pass down their experience and knowledge to their kin. Justin Congdon, Stanley Rapoport, Hillary Kaplan, Caleb Finch and Yves Christen deal with these aspects in as many chapters.

If brain size and longevity seem to have evolved in parallel, what respective influence do they still have on contemporary human populations? The exceptional rediscovery of IQ tests performed on Scottish children born in 1921 and the study of the survival of this cohort suggest a strong link between intelligence and survival. More classic studies on twins, on cohorts of elderly people or specific cohorts confirm these links as well as the connection with education level. The risk of Alzheimer's disease is known to increase greatly with age after 85 years. Nevertheless, the prevalence of dementia observed in centenarians or supercentenarians (age 110 and over) is much less than expected. These aspects are developed in a second part of the book by Ian Deary, Heiner Maier, Jean-François Dartigues, Howard Friedman, Gillis Samulson, Jean-Marie Robine and Carol Jagger. Dementia no longer appears to be inevitably linked to age. This is very good news in many countries, like France, where the number of centenarians will double in less than 10 years!

October 2002

JEAN-MARIE ROBINE
CALEB FINCH
YVES CHRISTEN

Contents

List of Contributors

Chêne, G.
Unité INSERM 330, Université de Bordeaux II, 146, rue Léo Saignat, 33076 Bordeaux cedex, France

Christen, Y.
Fondation Ipsen, 24, rue Erlanger, 75016 Paris, France

Christensen, K.
Institute of Public Health, University of Southern Denmark, Sdr. Boulevard 23 A, DK-5000 Odense C, Denmark

Congdon, J.D.
Savannah River Ecology Laboratory, Drawer E, Aiken, SC 29802, USA

Dartigues, J.F.
Unité INSERM 330, Université V. Segalen Bordeaux II, 146, rue Léo Saignat, 33076 Bordeaux cedex, France

Deary, I.J.
Department of Psychology, University of Edinburgh, 7 George Square, Edinburgh EH8 9JZ, Scotland, UK

Dehlin, O.
University Hospital MAS, Department of geriatrics, S-205 02 Malmö, Sweden

Finch, C.E.
Division of Neurogerontology, Ethel Percy Andrus Gerontology Center, University Park, MC-0191 3715 Mc Clintok, Los Angeles, CA 90089-0191, USA

Friedman, H.S.
Department of Psychology – 075, University of California, Riverside, CA 92521-0426, USA

Hagberg, B.
Gerontology Research Centre, Karl XII gatan 1, S-222 20 Lund, Sweden

Helmer, C.
Unité INSERM 330, Université de Bordeaux II, 146 rue Leo Saignat,
33076 Bordeaux cedex, France

Jagger, C.
University of Leicester, Department of Epidemiology and Public Health,
2228 Princess Road West, LEI 6TP Leicester, UK

Kaplan, H.S.
Department of Anthropology, University of New Mexico, Albuquerque,
NM 87131, USA

Kinney, O.M.
Darlington School, 1014 Cave Spring Road, Rome, GA 30161, USA

Letenneur, L.
Unité INSERM 330, Université de Bordeaux II, 146 rue Leo Saignat,
33076 Bordeaux cedex, France

Lewden, Ch.
Unité INSERM 330, Université de Bordeaux II, 146 rue Leo Saignat,
33076 Bordeaux cedex, France

Maier, H.
Max Planck Institute for Demographic Research, Doberaner Str. 114,
18057 Rostock, Germany

Markey, Ch.N.
Department of Psychology 075, University of California, Riverside,
CA 92521-0426, USA

McGue, M.
Department of Psychology, University of Minnesota, 75 East River road,
Minneapolis MN 55455, USA

Nagle, R.D.
Environmental Science and Studies, Juniata College, Huntingdon, PA 16652,
USA

Osentoski, M.F.
Department of Biology, University of Miami, 1301 Memorial Drive,
Coral Gables, Florida 33124, USA

Rapoport, S.I.
Laboratory of neurosciences, Institute of Aging, Building 10, Room 6C 103,
National, Rockville Pike, Bethesda, MD 20892, USA

Robine, J.-M.
INSERM, Equipe Démographie et Santé, Centre Val d'aurelle, Parc
Euromédecine, 34298 Montpellier cedex 5, France

Samuelsson, G.
Gerontology Research Center, Karl XII gatan 1, S-222 20 Lund, Sweden

Stanford, C.
Andrus Gerontology Center, Department of Biological Sciences, and
Department of Anthropology, University Park, MC-0191 3715 Mc Clintok,
Los Angeles, CA 90089-0191, USA

Starr, J.M.
Department of Geriatric Medicine, Royal Victoria Hospital, Craigleith Road,
Edinburgh EH4 2DN, Scotland, UK

Sundström, G.
Institute of Gerontology, Box 1038, S-551 11 Jönköping, Sweden

van Loben Sels, R.C.
Red Mountain High School, 7301 East Brown Road, Mesa, 85207 Arizona,
USA

Vaupel, J.W.
Max Planck Institute for Demographic Research, Doberaner Str. 114,
18057 Rostock, Germany

Whalley, L.J.
Department of Mental Health, University of Aberdeen, Clinical Research
Centre, Cornhill Hospital, Aberdeen AB25 2ZH, Scotland, UK

Time and Longevity: An Explanation of the Gap Between Genes and Brains?

Y. *Christen*

Summary

Humans have a brain three to four times larger than that of great apes and they live twice as long. The nervous system's role in regulating longevity links these two characteristics. The considerable expansion of the brain and a developmental change, itself linked to increased longevity, could have occurred relatively recently during human evolution, after the appearance of *Homo erectus* or *Homo ergaster*. These changes, as well as the neotenic character of the human species, seem to be linked to dietary changes: together they have exerted considerable influence on the social and cultural life of *Homo sapiens*.

Introduction

A Martian zoologist studying fauna, especially mammals, on Earth could not help but note the singularity of the species we call *Homo sapiens:* it has both a large brain (three to four times bigger than that of our nearest cousins in nature, the apes) and a long life span (twice that of apes). We note that these two characteristics are extremely variable in nature, even within the primate order: small lemurs such as the mouse lemur *(Microcebus)* or the tree shrew (Tupaia) live one sixth as long as humans and have a brain 300 times smaller (but brain weight varies much less than body weight: the gorilla is about 1000 times larger than a mouse lemur but has a brain "only" 100 times larger). These variations go together with spectacular differences in the timing of life history events: a female mouse lemur might leave 10 million descendants before the gorilla reaches sexually maturity! These parameters thus vary greatly by phenotype. Our extraterrestrial should thus wonder, logically, if the genetic variation within primates is equally great. If he knew how to gain access to our scientific literature, or at least the issues of *Nature* and *Science* from February 2001, he would also learn most of what he needs to know about the decoding of the human genome. And he might be astonished to learn that a species with two highly complex attributes (a brain that is not only large but contains an incredible number of synapses, and an exceptional longevity) is not any more genetically complex than a mouse, and not even extraordinary compared with a fruit fly or a worm *(Caenorhabditis elegans)*. Our hypothetical Martian would have every reason to wonder about how to interpret all of these data together.

Finch et al. (Eds.)
Brain and Longevity
© Springer-Verlag Berlin Heidelberg 2003

Brain and Longevity: Evolution

The recent decoding of the human genome has led to a downward revision of the estimated number of genes possessed by *Homo sapiens*. The public project assessed this number at 31 000, the Celera project at 26 000, and the final count will probably end up at between 30 000 and 40 000. Mice have a similar number of genes, *Drosophila* have on the order of 13 000, *C. elegans* 18 000, and a plant 26 000.

Thus the genetic complexity of humans does not clearly differentiate us from other species. From one point of view, this is hardly surprising: all contemporary living creatures have the same evolutionary seniority and are therefore also roughly equally complex.

Humans nonetheless present elements of particular complexity, especially, the volume of their brain and their exceptional longevity. Moreover, these two criteria are associated in the living world. George Sacher called the brain "the organ of longevity" (Sacher 1962) and suggested that it serves as a pacemaker for embryo growth. The confirmation of this theory, originally proposed for mammals, suggest in other, very different phyla a relation of some kind between neuronal function and longevity. In particular, Wolkow et al. (2000) report an insulin-like regulation by the nervous system in *C. elegans;* this finding points to the nervous system as a central regulator of animal longevity. Similar findings have been obtained in *Drosophila:* life span is extended with the loss of CHICO, a gene that encodes an insulin-receptor substrate that functions in an insulin/insulin-like growth factor signaling pathway (Clancy et al. 2001).

Sacher (1997) established a formula for the relation between life span and brain weight in the mammal phylum: maximum possible longevity (years) = 10.8 brain weight (g) × 0.633 body weight (g) –0.225.

Table 1 illustrates the simultaneous evolution of brain weight and maximum life span, as observed empirically and as calculated by this type of for-

Table 1. The evolution of brain, body weight and maximum life span[a]

Common name	Cranial capacity (cm^3)	Body weight (g)	Maximum lifespan potential (years) observed	predicted
tupaïa (tree shrew)	4.3	275	7	7.7
marmoset	9.8	413	15	12
squirrel monkey	24.8	630	21	20
rhesus monkey	106	8 719	29	27
baboon	179	16 000	36	33
gibbon	104	5 500	32	30
orangutan	420	69 000	60	41
gorilla	550	140 000	40	42
chimpanzee	410	49 000	45	43
human	1 446	65 000	95	92

[a] From Cutler 1985 (with permission)

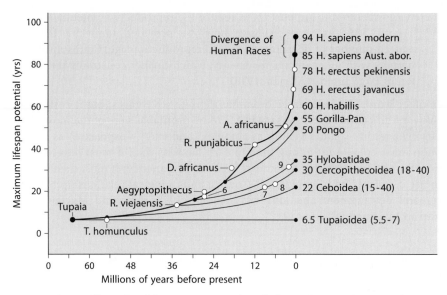

Fig. 1. Evolution of longevity of the primate species along the hominid-ancestral sequence leading to humans. Open circles: extinct species. Closed circles: living species. dating. (From Cutler 1985, with permission)

mula. The almost identical tracings of the evolution of each characteristic are surprising. In fact, when we consider the evolution of the human phylum, we are struck by the rapidity with which these two characteristics appear to have evolved over the past four million years (Fig. 1; but the data on the maximum longevity of prehuman and human fossil species must be considered cautiously; although the mean life span of the latter is thought to have been on the order of that of apes, this assessment does not exclude the possibility of some very long lives). Nevertheless, several caveats ought to be noted about these correlations with life span: they are only statistically formulated and they do not require a link between the variables (Finch 1990). Moreover, brain weight curiously appears to have decreased over recent millennia (the Neanderthal's brain was heavier than ours; Ruff et al. 1997), and gerontologists thought until recently that maximum life span had also reached a ceiling. This viewpoint, however, has been challenged by recent studies on longevity in Sweden (Wilmoth et al. 2000) and on supercentenarians (Robine 2001).

We might be surprised by this human singularity, but the explanation is clear, as John Allman notes:

> Animals with big brains are rare. If brains enable animals to adapt to changing environments, why is it that so few animals have large brains? The reason is that big brains are very expensive, costly in term of time, energy and anatomical complexity. Large brains take a long time to mature, and consequently large-brained animals are dependent on their parents for a long time. The slow development of large-brained offspring and the extra

energy required to support them reduce the reproductive potentials of the parents. Thus extra-special care must be provided to insure that the reduced number of offspring survive to reproduction age. Brains must also compete with other organs for energy, which further constrains the evolution of large brains (Allman, 1998).

In other words, having a large brain has definite advantages, but it costs a lot: some modifications are necessary if it is to be profitable. One of the most obvious involves life span: a factory as complex (and energy-expensive) as a large brain must operate for a long time to earn back its cost. It must have enough time for optimal training, to increase its learning capacity; it must then be able to use its talents for a long period. There is thus a logical relationship between cerebral development and longevity (Allman 1998; Rose and Mueller 1998; Kaplan this volume).

Longevity, Development and "Life-History" Features

Longevity is not an independent biological criterion but is directly associated with delayed development. The naturalist Buffon noted more than two centuries ago:

> la durée totale de la vie peut se mesurer en quelque façon par celle du temps de l'accroissement; un arbre ou un animal qui prend en peu de temps tout son accroissement périt beaucoup plus tôt qu'un arbre auquel il faut plus de temps pour croître [...] L'homme qui met trente ans à croître vit quatre-vingts ou cent ans; le chien qui ne croît que pendant deux ou trois ans, ne vit que dix ou douze ans
> ([total life span can in some way be measured by the duration of the growth period; a tree or an animal that is rapidly fully grown perishes much earlier than a tree, which needs more time to grow [...] Humans who spent thirty years growing up live for eighty or one hundred years; the dog who only grows for two or three years only lives for ten or twelve.] Buffon 1707–1788).

In *Drosophila*, increased life span is correlated with a later onset of reproductive capability (Rose 1991); in *C. elegans* a mutation that slows the growth of the germ line may simultaneously slow the animal's rate of aging, enabling it to remain youthful longer to have progeny (Hsin and Kenyon 1999). There is evidence of trade-offs between longevity and fertility (Kirkwood and Westendorp 2000). Life span is associated with a set of "life-history" features linked to development, including delayed reproduction and prolonged childhood. Both these features are characteristics of humans in comparison with other primates (Harvey and Clutton-Brock 1985). The entire maturation process is thus modified and numerous consequences ensue – related to family and social life and to the appearance of culture. There is a higher probability that some individuals will live to become old: these may have an important social and cultural role, clearly visible among humans but also identifiable in others with a long life span, in particular elephants, among whom the crucial role played by matriarchs in the transmission of knowledge has been recognized (McComb et al. 2001). The long life span of humans also involves a long menopause – a ubiquitous phenomenon in female mammals (Finch and Sapolsky 1999), but particularly long in humans (Madame Calment lived 70–80 years after menopause!). This fact reinforces the controversial "grandmother hypothesis" (Sherman 1998) according to which menopause is an adaptation that enables old women to nurture their grandchildren.

Extended longevity presupposes the existence of education and of social life, which together protect the young during their formative period; they also protect the adult and the elderly and promote the exchange of information at all ages, thereby optimizing the potential of the cerebral machine we call the brain. From the point of view of energy, we note that men and women differ in both brain weight and longevity. Allman and Hasenstaub (1999, 2000) have proposed an interesting hypothesis on this subject: the difference in longevity between the sexes may be a function of the pattern of parental care. When we look at a table of primates that reports the life span of both sexes and participation in parental care, we see that the parent in charge of child care lives longer (Table 2). This parent is most often the female, at least among the great apes. But in several small New World monkeys, such as the Titi *(Callicebus)* and Owl *(Aotus)* monkeys, it is the male who is responsible for this task and it is he who lives longer. The comparison between two similar lesser apes, the gibbon and the siamang, is still more astonishing. Gibbons lives in pairs but the father plays no direct role in the offspring's life, while siamang fathers carry the babies during their second year of life. Female gibbons live substantially longer than the males, but female siamangs do not. Caretaking is itself inversely associated with risk-seeking, insofar as the sex not responsible for parenting will naturally be

Table 2. The ratio of male to female life span and patterns of parental care for primates. The male/female weight ratio is an index of sexual dimorphism[a]

Primate	Male/female Survival ratio	Male care		Male/Female Weight ratio
Titi monkey	1.208	Carries infant from birth	↑	1.139
Owl monkey	1.151	Carries infant from birth		1.026
Siamang	1.093	Carries infant in second year		1.279
Goeldi's monkey	1.027	Both parents carry infant	Increasing Male Survival — Increasing Male Care	1.000
Human (Sweden 1780–1991)	0.924–0.951	Supports economically, some care		1.182
Gorilla	0.889	Protects, plays with offspring		1.851
Gibbon	0.834	Pair-living, but little direct role		1.044
Orangutan	0.831	None		2.095
Spider monkey	0.786	Rare or negligible		1.001
Chimpanzee	0.667	Rare or negligible		1.355

[a] From Allman and Hasenstaub 2000

the one who spends the most time exploring new resources, a necessary task in a constantly changing environment and an activity necessarily more dangerous than routine.

The Advancement of the Developmental Timetable in Humans

The general idea according to which longevity results from life-history trade-offs (Kirkwood and Westendorp 2000) applies to the case of the developmental modifications that accompany the long duration of human life and the cerebral development that goes with it. In this case, the cost results directly from the risk of dying before the reproductive period and from the long interval between births that is so serious a risk for species with long life spans. It is probably for this reason that the developmental delays of *Homo sapiens* are less than they might be as a function of brain weight. Allman (1998) showed a linear relationship in diverse primate species between brain weight and several developmental parameters, including appearance of the first and second molars and of the wisdom-teeth, sexual maturity, and life span. Curiously, for each of these stages of maturation except the last, humans develop earlier than expected. Based on curves representing the overall order of primates, Allman calculated the theoretical dates of these events and compared them to those actually observed. The first molar should appear at 19.3 years but actually appears at 6.4 years, the second molar at 29.2 years compared with 11.1 in reality, wisdom teeth at 37.8 years rather than at 20.5, and sexual maturity at 44.5 years instead of at 16.6. Only the length of the maximum life span seems fairly consistent with reality: 101.5 years in theory against 105 (in Allman's assessment). Thus the entire developmental timetable is advanced in humans. Allman (1998) deduces from this that "if the brain is the pacemaker for development, humans have accelerated maturation relative to what would be expected for a primate of our brain size."

This observation should be compared with the older theory of Louis Bolk, the Dutch anatomist (1926), about the pedomorphic character of the human species (Bolk used the term fetalization; pedomorphosis is a term designating the retention of youthful ancestral features by adults; the word neoteny involves the retardation of somatic development and differs from progenesis, or precocious sexual maturation; in the old literature, however, neoteny means the capacity to reproduce as a larva, like the axolotl, a larva of the salamander of the genus *Ambystoma*). Our skull and our brain are more similar to those of a great ape fetus than to those of an adult of the same species (Starck and Kummer 1992; Fig. 2). For this reason, Bolk suggested that humans are neotenic animals, capable of reproducing at a larval (or fetal) stage; this explains their delayed development and their morphology. This capacity to reproduce while immature, thus to mature slowly in absolute terms but at a relatively accelerated rate from the point of view of cerebral volume, may be a consequence of the biological constraint associated with development that is too late, that is, the risk of a

A   B

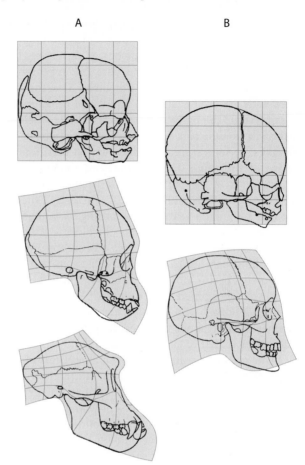

Fig. 2. Comparative cranial ontogeny of chimpanzee (A) and human (B) using transformed coordinate analysis. Despite similar fetal beginning and similar direction of transformation, the adult human skull clearly differs from the adult ape skull but departs far less from the juvenile form

considerable biological investment that would be for naught, if death preceded reproduction.

Despite its age and even though many of its elements have been rejected, Bolk's theory still holds some interest. As Gould has pointed out, "I believe that human beings are 'essentially' neotenous, not because I can enumerate a list of important pedomorphic features, but because a *general, temporal retardation of development has clearly characterized human evolution. This retardation established a matrix within which all trends in the evolution of human morphology must be assessed*" (Gould 1977). Several authors have already suggested that the genes involved in this neoteny may be those most characteristic of the human species and predicted that a comparison of the genomes of humans and chimpanzees would make it possible to identify or even to manipulate these genes in order to increase longevity further (Cutler 1986). Cutler (1986) thus envisaged the appearance of a still more neotenic *Homo futurus* who would live for 600 years but not attain sexual maturity until the age of 90!

When Did the Brain and Longevity Become Hominized?

If its development, neotenic or not, is the aspect most characteristic of *Homo sapiens*, then it is essential to date the appearance during evolution of any changes in its developmental timetable. Alas, the "life-history" features associated with the prolongation of childhood or delayed reproduction do not leave fossil traces. The brain too leaves few direct traces, but fossil skulls help us to assess its volume as a function of skull volume as well as by several anatomic features. Serious arguments thus suggest that *Homo habilis* (the first representative of the genus *Homo*) possessed linguistic capabilities, judging by the enlargement of the portion of the frontal lobe corresponding to Broca's area (Tobias 1995). Paleoanthropologists currently believe that at this stage (between 2.3 and 1.8 million years ago, according to various assessments) these primates (but not the contemporaneous – or older – *Australopithecus*) took a decisive step towards hominization. *Homo erectus* and *Homo ergaster* (between 1.9 and 0.8 million years ago) are thought to have moved further towards hominization by evolving brains much more like ours. But when might a major change in the timing of development have occurred? We know of some Hominidae fossils that show individuals who seem to have lived well past simple maturity, but this teaches us little about their real longevity, which we suppose to be essentially equivalent to that of current apes.

One possible means of studying the process of maturation in primate fossils involves teeth – their eruption, growth, and structure, mainly in the enamel (found on the crowns) and the dentine (the internal hard tissue). This method can be used on the fossil remains of young hominids, either directly or by computed tomography scans. A first set of data led to the conclusion that *H. habilis* had a pattern of tooth development similar to that of *Australopithecus*, while *H. erectus* and *H. ergaster* shared similarities with modern humans (Moggi-Cecchi 2001). A more recent study by Dean et al. (2001) yielded different results. It showed that, in terms of enamel-formation rates and crown-formation times, *Australopithecus*, an early representatives of the genus *Homo* – *H. habilis*, including the famous "Turkana boy" (an almost complete specimen), and *H. erectus* – resembled modern and fossil apes more closely than they do modern humans. This result is intriguing because we often consider *H. erectus* and *H. ergaster* as real humans, because of their posture, body size and limb proportion. Their cerebral volume, however, was closer to that of *Australopithecus* and *H. habilis*. As D. Moggi-Cecchi has suggested, "it seems that the human brain and body structural evolved in a mosaic pattern, with human-like rates of dental development and a marked increase in relative brain size apparently occurring later than other humanlike body structures" (Moggi-Cecchi 2001 b). On the other hand, we note that Neanderthal Man, today excluded from the phylum of modern humans despite his very voluminous brain, had the modern human structure of enamel growth. All this provides spectacular confirmation of the importance of the relationship between cerebral volume and the processes of maturation and therefore, probably, longevity. Moreover, it seems probable from this point of view that the most important modifications associated with development and maturation in hominid evolution occurred after the appearance of *H. erectus*, that is, relatively recently in human evolution.

Although it remains difficult to date the appearance of any crucial mutation in the course of hominization (or even to be certain of its existence), we can suppose that it might have been related to changes in the environment and diet of the ancient hominids (Kelley 2001). Finch and Stanford (this volume) hypothesize that the appearance of the epsilon 3 allele of the gene coding for apolipoprotein E (apo E) played an important role in increasing longevity (great apes possess only the E4 allele, which is overrepresented in the population of persons with Alzheimer's disease and underrepresented in centenarians) together with a change in diet corresponding to the period when *H. erectus* became carnivorous. The experimental data reveal that the E3 and E2 isoforms of apo E affect the growth of neurites more significantly than does E4. Their appearance must therefore have had important functional consequences associated with a better use of cholesterol at the neuron level. The appearance of sporadic mutations leading to apo E3 may have also been selected in humans in relation to the enormous brain expansion, delayed maturation, and increasing duration of postnatal care (Finch and Sapolsky 1999). This hypothesis posits that a crucial genetic event occurred at the stage of *H. erectus*, perhaps when prehistoric humans first discovered or began the generalized use of fire.

It is nonetheless difficult to see the onset of this mutation as the essential element of hominization, since many humans have no E2 or E3 allele (but these subjects, homozygotes for E4, are at high risk of developing Alzheimer's disease), a fact implying that the E4 allele presents advantages in specific conditions. In any case, the dietary change linked to the increased hunting by the ancestors of *H. sapiens* can reasonably be seen as a decisive element in its evolution, as shown by the comparative analysis of today's hunter-gatherer populations and chimpanzees (Kaplan et al. 2000). Kaplan et al. (2000; and this volume) proposed that the shift to calorie-dense, large-package, skill-intensive food resources is responsible for the unique evolutionary trajectory of the genus *Homo*. This shift would have produced co-evolutionary selection pressures that, in turn, operated to produce the extreme intelligence, long developmental period, three-generational system of resource flows, and exceptionally long adult life that are characteristic of our species.

The Burden of the Old Brain

With both a voluminous brain and substantial longevity, *H. sapiens* combines two risk factors for cerebral fragility. It has generally been accepted that the central nervous system neurons are post-mitotic cells that stop multiplying shortly after birth, so that the longevity of individuals is also that of their brain neurons (Rakic 1985). The discovery of stem cells in the brain, even in mammals, including humans and even aged humans, suggests that this "dogma" is less absolute than previously thought (Gage 2000). It is nonetheless true that the neocortex neuron network in primates is composed nearly entirely (or even completely, according to Kornack and Rakic 2001) of cells that survive throughout an individual's life. Our neurons are often considered to be as old as we are: "a 75-year-old individual has 75-year-old neurons" (Rakic 1998). They therefore must cope with multiple aggressions, in the form of ischemic accidents or neurodegenerative diseases. Alzheimer's disease is the most common of these diseases: it is remarkable that it is essentially characteristic of the human species, although its existence in apes and other mammals is debated (Finch and Stanford, this volume). Rapoport (1988) thinks that this particular disease affects only areas of the cerebral cortex (association areas) that are developed primarily in humans.

In general, the brain's sensitivity to disease processes is attributed to its relative stability; accordingly, in principle, plasticity of the processes related to these phenomena would be beneficial. We can thus imagine, with Mesulam (1999), that Alzheimer's disease might result not only from a degenerative phenomenon but also from the deficit of counterbalancing plastic repair processes. Nonetheless we can consider that the relative stability of the neuron network in the adult cortex is functionally useful, especially in species with a long life span. As Rakic stressed (1985), "one can speculate that a prolonged period of interaction with the environment, as pronounced as it is in all primates, especially humans, requires a stable set of neurons to retain acquired experiences in the pattern of their synaptic connectivity." It is therefore conceivable that a disease such as Alzheimer's involves not insufficient plasticity but a pathological plasticity likely to account for the modification of the neuron network involved in recall and therefore the memory problems of subjects with dementia. The fact that a signaling system such as Notch, involved in embryo formation, may also act in the adult brain to limit neurogenesis (Sestan and Rakic 2002) argues in favor of this hypothesis, an argument reinforced more generally by the relationship between the presenilins associated with Alzheimer's disease and the Notch system (De Strooper et al. 2002)

It is not surprising that the brain, built to last a long time, might be the target of particular diseases associated with the loss of neurons and, perhaps even more important, of synapses (Terry and Katzman 2001). The prolongation of the life span suggests that the number of these diseases will increase in the future. It is also expected that their frequency, especially that of Alzheimer's disease, will depend on the cerebral reserve (Mortimer 1995), with no defect visible until after a critical level of neuronal connections is lost. This level will be reached more quickly when the cerebral reserve is lowest. In this regard, we note that epidemiologic observations and studies of populations for whom we know the youthful IQ suggest that the risk of Alzheimer's disease is lower in people with larger brains (estimated indirectly by head circumference; Graves et al. 2001), in those with a high level of education (Dartigues et al. this volume), and in those with an elevated cognitive capacity during childhood (Whalley et al. 2000). They also show that the most intellectually gifted subjects tend to live longer (Deary et al. this volume; Friedman and Markey, this volume) and that cognitive impairment is associated with an increased risk of death (Maier et al. this volume), again confirming the existence of a relationship between the brain and longevity.

Time Is of the Essence

Biology most often studies coding systems (the genotype) and the structures that result from them (the phenotype). Generally speaking, the development of a genotype during an individual's life is studied less, even though everyone agrees on the importance to be attributed to the process of epigenesis. Phenotypes are frequently interpreted as a means by which environmental (extrinsic) factors intervene in the expression of the genetic message. It is equally essential to stress that development involves a chronological activation of the genetic message and that the history of the species and the individual depends on the speed with which this occurs. As Kennedy and Dehay (1993) have shown, cortical development is more usefully thought of in terms of the timing of specification events rather than as a balance between intrinsic (genetic) and extrinsic control. Time is an essential factor in ontogenesis as it is in phylogenesis. In this context, factors of genetic regulation such as transcription factors probably play an essential role in explaining how a relatively small number of genes may allow the formation of a synaptic network that is several orders of magnitude larger (Changeux 2001). These systems appear to intervene in a rhythm of development peculiar to humans and thus explain its neotenic character. The number of genes is probably not the most important element in this regard, as Baltimore (2001) points out:

> it is clear that we do not gain our undoubted complexity over worms and plants by using many more genes. Understanding what does give us our complexity – our enormous behavioral repertoire, ability to produce conscious action, remarkable physical coordination (shared with other vertebrates), precisely tuned alterations in response to external variations of the environment, learning memory... need I go on? – remains a challenge for the future.

A comparative study of animal genomes, of chimpanzees and humans in particular, will undoubtedly provide interesting information. Nonetheless we may doubt, along with Baltimore (2001), that we will find an explanation there of the origin of language, abstract reasoning or thumb opposition to the other fingers, especially since our genomes seem very similar. The demonstration by Lai et al. (2001) of the first gene associated with human language (FOXP2) will make this type of comparative analysis possible. Very similar genetic sequences have been identified in mice, monkeys and apes but recent data shown that human FOXP2 contains changes in amino-acid coding and a pattern of nucleotide polymorphism, which strongly suggest that this gene has been the target of selection during the last 200 000 years of human evolution (Enard et al. 2002). More generally, Svante Pääbo (2001) has predicted that "when the chimpanzee genome sequences become available, we are sure to find that its gene contents and organization are very similar (if not identical) to our own." It is therefore probable that the essential differences will not be found in genes for structures, which are relatively easy for computers to compare, but in those for regulatory systems. The hypothesis we propose here is that: 1)° the differences between *H. sapiens* and apes are less than we, with our anthropocentric viewpoint, tend to think; and 2)° they may be explained by the neotenic aspects of our species, which in turn are associated with changes at the level of transcription factors rather than one or several specific mutations of genes for structures. In this case, the most humanizing genetic events would directly concern developmental timing, which is at the origin of both our extremely high encephalization quotients and our exceptional longevity. Time is not a reality that monopolizes us from the outside. It is not an extrinsic factor but an essential element that contributes to the very definition of our species.

References

Allman J (1998) Evolving brains. Scientific American Library, New York

Allman J, Hasenstaub A (1999) Brains, maturation times, and parenting. Neurobiol Aging 20: 447–454

Allman J, Hasenstaub A (2000) Caretaking, risk-seeking, and survival in anthropoid primates. In: Robine J-M, Kirkwood TBL, Allard M (Eds) Sex and longevity: sexuality, gender, reproduction, parenthood. Springer, Heidelberg, pp 75–89

Baltimore D (2001) Our genome unveiled. Nature 409: 814–816

Bolk L (1926) Das Problem der Menschwerdung. Gustav Fischer, Jena

Buffon (Leclerc GL, comte de) (1749–1804) Histoire naturelle, générale et particulière. Imprimerie Royale, Paris, 1749–1804, vol. 2

Changeux JP (2001) The non-linear evolution of brain-genome complexity from mouse to man. Lecture for the Colloque Médecine et Recherche, Fondation Ipsen on Neurosciences in the postgenomic era.

Clancy DJ, Gems D, Harshamn LG, Oldham S, Stocker H, Hafen E, Leevers SJ, Partridge L (2001) Extension of life-span by loss of CHICO, a *Drosophila* insulin receptor substrate protein. Science 292: 104–106.

Cutler RG (1985) Biology of aging and longevity. Gerontol Biomed Acta 1: 35–61

Cutler R (1986) Interview. Omni 9 (n° 1): 109–114, 174–181

Dean C, Leakey MG, Reid D, Schrenk F, Schwartz GT, Stringer C, Walker A (2001) Growth processes in teeth distinguish modern humans from *Homo erectus* and earlier hominins. Nature 414: 628–631

De Strooper B, Israël A, Checler F, Christen Y eds (2002) Notch from neurodevelopment to neurodegeneration: keeping the fate. Springer, Heidelberg

Enard W, Przeworski M, Fisher S, Lai CSL, Wiebe V, Kitano T, Monaco AP, Pääbo S (2002) Molecular evolution of *FOXP2*, a gene involved in speech and language. Nature 418: 869–872

Finch CE (1990) Longevity, senescence, and the genome. Chicago University Press, Chicago.

Finch CE, Sapolsky RM (1999) The evolution of Alzheimer disease, the reproductive schedule and apoE isoforms. Neurobiol Aging 20: 407–428

Gage FH (2000) Mammalian neural stem cells. Science 287: 1433–1438.

Gould SJ (1977) Ontogeny and phylogeny. Harvard University Press, Cambridge, MA

Graves AB, Mortimer JA, Bowen JD, McCormick WC, McCurry SM, Schellenberg GD, Larson EB (2001) Head circumference and incident Alzheimer's disease. Modification by apolipoprotein E. Neurology 57: 1453–1460

Harvey PH, Clutton-Brock TH (1985) Life history variation in primates. Evolution 39: 559–581

Hsin H, Kenyon C (1999) Signals from the reproductive system regulate the lifespan of *C. elegans*. Nature 399: 362–366.

Kaplan H, Hill K, Lancaster J, Hurtado AM (2000) A theory of human life history evolution: diet, intelligence, and longevity. Evol Anthropol 9: 156–185.

Kelley J (2001) Enamel microstructure in hominids: New characteristics for a new paradigm. In: Minugh-Purvis N, McNamara KJ (Eds.) Human evolution through developmental change. Johns Hopkins Univ Press, Baltimore, 319–348

Kennedy H, Dehay C (1993) The importance of developmental timing in cortical specification. Perpect Dev Neurobiol 1: 93–99

Kirkwood TBL, Westendorps RGJ (2000) Human longevity at the cost of reproductive success: trade-offs in the life history. In: Robine J-M, Kirkwood TBL, Allard M (eds) Sex and longevity: sexuality, gender, reproduction, parenthood. Springer, Heidelberg, pp 1–6

Kornack DR, Rakic P (2001) Cell proliferation without neurogenesis in adult primate neocortex. Science 294: 2127–2130

Lai CSL, Fisher SE, Hurst JA, Vargha-Khadem F, Monaco AP (2001) A forkhead-domain gene is mutated in a severe speech and language disorder. Nature 413: 519–523

McComb K, Moss C, Durant SM, Baker L, Sayialel S (2001) Matriarchs as repositories of social knowledge in African elephants. Science 292: 491–494

Mesulam MM (1999) Neuroplasticity failure in Alzheimer's disease: bridging the gap between plaques and tangles. Neuron 24: 531–529

Moggi-Cecchi J (2001 a) Pattern of dental development of Australopithecus africanus, with some inference on their evolution and the origin of the genus Homo. In: Tobias PV, Raath MA, Moggi-Cecchi J, Doyle GA (eds) Humanity from African naissance to coming millennia. Firenze Univ Press, Florence & Witwatersrand Univ. Press, Johannesburg, pp 125–134

Moggi-Cecchi J (2001 b) Questions of growth. Nature 414: 595–597

Mortimer JA (1995) The continuum hypothesis of Alzheimer's disease and normal aging: the role of brain reserve. Alzheimers Res 1: 67–70

Pääbo S (2001) The human genome and our view of ourselves. Science 291: 1219–1220

Rakic P (1985) Limits of neurogenesis in primates. Science 227: 1054–1056

Rakic P (1998) Young neurons for old brains? Nat Neurosci 1: 645–647

Rapoport SI (1988) A phylogenetic hypothesis for Alzheimer's disease. In: Sinet P-M, Lamour Y, Christen Y (eds) Genetics and Alzheimer's disease. Springer Verlag, Heidelberg, pp. 62–88

Robine J-M (2001) A new biodemographic model to explain the trajectory of mortality. Exp Gerontol 36: 899–914

Rose M (1991) Evolutionary biology of aging. Oxford University Press, New York

Rose M, Mueller LD (1998) Evolution of the human lifespan: past, future and present. Am J Human Biol 10: 409–420

Ruff C, Trinkaus E, Holliday T (1997) Body mass and encephalization in Pleistocene Homo. Nature 387: 173–176

Sacher GA (1962) The role of physiological fluctuations in the aging process and the relation of longevity to the size of the central nervous system. In: Brues AM, Sacher GA (eds) Aging and levels of biological organization. University of Chicago Press, Chicago, p. 266

Sacher GA (1977): Life table modification and life prolongation. In: Finch CE, Hayflick L (eds) Handbook of the biology and aging. Van Nostrand Reinhold, New York, vol I, pp 582–638

Sestan N, Rakic P (2002) Notch signaling in the brain: more than just a developmental story. In: De Strooper B, Israël A, Checler F, Christen Y eds: Notch from neurodevelopment to neurodegeneration: keeping the fate. Springer, Heidelberg, 19–40.

Sherman PW (1998) The evolution of menopause. Nature 392: 759–761

Starck D, Kummer B (1962) Zur Ontogenese des Schimpansenschädels. Anthrop Anz 25: 204–215

Terry RD, Katzman R (2001) Life span and synapses: will there be a primary senile dementia? Neurobiol Aging 22: 347–348

Tobias PV (1995) The communication of the dead. Earliest vestiges of the origin of articulate language. Nederlands Museum voor Anthropologie en Praehistorie.

Whalley LJ, Starr JM, Athawes R, Hunter D, Pattie A, Deary IJ (2000) Childhood mental ability and dementia. Neurology 28: 1455–1459

Wilmoth JR, Deegan LJ, Lundström H, Horiuchi S (2000) Increase of maximum life-span in Sweden, 1861–1999. Science 289: 2366–2368

Wolkow CA, Kimura KD, Lee M-S, Ruvkun G (2000) Regulation of *C. elegans* life-span by insulinlike signaling in the nervous system. Science 290: 147–150

Life History and Demographic Aspects of Aging in the Long-Lived Turtle *(Emydoidea blandingii)*

J. D. Congdon, R. D. Nagle, M. F. Osentoski, O. M. Kinney and R. C. van Loben Sels

Introduction

More than 40 years ago Williams (1957) asked, "Why is it that after achieving the seemingly miraculous feat of morphogenesis, a complex metazoan is unable to perform the apparently much simpler task of merely maintaining that which is already formed?" Answering that question remains central to understanding the evolution of life histories in general, and aging and longevity specifically. The preponderance of relatively short-compared to long-lived organisms suggests that morphogenesis is easier to accomplish than is maintenance of soma, whereas the broad range of longevities of organisms (Finch 1999) demonstrates that maintaining soma for extended periods of time is possible. The underlying assumption of the "disposable soma" theory of aging (Kirkwood 1999) is that the expense of maintaining the immortal germ cells is always warranted, whereas investing in maintaining somatic cells depends on their contribution to the welfare of the germ cells. Because the death of many individuals results from extrinsic factors (predators, disease, accidents), large investments in maintaining somatic cells are often not warrented. Kirkwood (1999) restated Williams' (1957) question to ask, "...how long do germ cells need soma to last?" From a life history perspective, the question becomes, under what environmental conditions can selection favor prolonged investment in maintenance of soma?

To initiate the process of natural selection for longer life span, germ cells have to be housed within individuals that for some reason begin to survive longer and as a result produce more successful copies of their germ cell lines. Because most organisms are killed before they become old, escape from the extrinsic sources of mortality may be the most important mechanism initiating selection for traits that extend longevity. Escape from extrinsic mortality can happen by chance (e.g., invasion of islands without predators) and with little or no additional costs to individuals. For example, an insular population of the gecko *Oplodactylus duvauceli* delayed sexual maturity and lived much longer than did a closely related species on the mainland (Barwick 1982). Escape from extrinsic mortality can also occur by altering behavior, body design, or both (e.g., flight, development of poisons or irritants, or armor), mechanisms that are often associated with substantial costs to individuals. Ultimately, benefits to the germ cell line that are derived through increased investments in maintenance of soma are all that is important.

Finch et al. (Eds.)
Brain and Longevity
© Springer-Verlag Berlin Heidelberg 2003

Once individuals begin to live longer, traits increasing the proportion of births late in life versus births early in life allow the selection of modifiers that reduce, prevent or postpone the expression of senescence traits (Medawar 1952; Williams 1957). The Relative Reproductive Rate hypothesis (Williams 1957; Congdon et al. 2001) predicts that, particularly in long-lived organisms, older individuals in a population should exhibit traits that increase the proportion of late to early births directly through: 1) reproductive output (e.g., clutch size, egg size, reproductive frequency, and total lifetime reproductions), 2) reproductive success (nest survivorship, parental investment), or 3) indirectly through increased survivorship of older adults, compared to younger individuals (Congdon et al. 2001).

Among vertebrates, body growth continues through adulthood in some taxa (indeterminate growth of amphibians and reptiles), whereas growth stops in some others (determinate growth of mammals and birds). Indeterminate growth is an obvious mechanism that directly couples age to increased body size, and among and within populations of reptiles, increased body size is almost always positively correlated with increased reproductive output (Congdon and Gibbons 1985) and may be associated with increased survival (Fox 1978; Sinervo et al. 1992; Janzen et al. 2000; Congdon et al. 1999; Bodie and Semlitsch. 2000). In contrast, individuals with determinant growth lack the direct mechanism of increasing adult body size that couples age to increased reproductive output. However, increased experience (i.e., learning) associated with age that results in reduced mortality or increased reproductive output in older individuals represents a mechanism for increasing the proportion of late to early births in organisms, regardless of adult growth patterns.

Contrasting Views of Aging

The most prevalent view of aging (senescence) is based primarily on data from mammals. In general, mammals accumulate physical and physiological traits that reduce performance, survivorship, and reproductive output in older individuals. The Senescence Hypothesis (Hamilton 1966; Williams 1966; Charlesworth 1995; Rose 1996) predicts that older individuals will have reduced survivorship or reproductive output compared to younger individuals in a population, a view that has by default been assumed to apply to reptiles.

Reproductive senescence has been suggested as a cause of reduced reproduction in older female turtles (Cagle 1944; Gibbons 1969; Legler 1960; Moll 1979). However, a review of reports of reproductive senescence indicated that individuals were categorized as old based on physical appearance and body size rather than on actual ages. In addition, most of the reports of reproductive senescence occurred before it had been documented that females skip reproduction in some years (Congdon and Gibbons 1990). A comparison of reproductive traits of young (known age) and old (known minimum ages of over 55 years) Blanding's turtles revealed no evidence for reduced reproductive output of the older females (Congdon and van Loben Sels 1993).

Age-specific traits related to reproduction and survival form the conceptual and theoretical basis of life history evolution (Cole 1954; Williams 1966). In general, a life history is a set of co-evolved traits (e.g., age-specific survivorship, reproductive output, and growth rates of juveniles and adults, age and body size at maturity, duration of lifetime reproduction, and overall longevity of adults). Not all combinations of traits can result in a stable population under a given set of environmental conditions; those combinations that do are called "feasible suites of traits or feasible demographies" (Dunham et al. 1989; Congdon et al. 1993). Because Gibbons' (1976) observation that the importance of aging in natural populations had not been demonstrated remains true today, the importance of understanding ecological and intrinsic factors linking age and aging to the evolution of feasible suites of life history traits remains a major focus of life history studies.

To life historians, turtles as a group represent the epitome of long-lived vertebrates (Wilbur and Morin 1988) and paragons of delayed sexual maturity, longevity, and iteroparity (repeated reproduction). Because it is among the longest-lived and most intensively studied freshwater turtles, Blanding's turtle is an excellent model for the study of evolution of life histories in general and for the evolution of longevity specifically. One population on the University of Michigan's E. S. George Reserve (ESGR) has been studied for 37 of the past 50 years [1953–1957 (Owen Sexton); 1968–1972 (Henry Wilbur), and 1975–2001 (present study)].

We examined the published and unpublished information that pertains to age, aging and longevity for the ESGR population of Blanding's turtles and reviewed the literature on ecological aspects of aging in turtles. We examined whether relationships between age and body size support indeterminate growth as a mechanism for the evolution of longevity, we reviewed reproductive data and survival of different age groups of female Blanding's turtles in relation to predictions based on the Relative Reproductive Rate and Senescence Hypotheses, and we summarized data from genetic determination of male parentage for evidence of age-specific reproductive success of males. The fact that older Blanding's turtle females reproduce more frequently than do younger females (Congdon et al. 2001) requires that older females also harvest more resources or allocate resources more efficiently than do younger females. Therefore, we examined data from the ESGR study for evidence that learning may contribute to how older Blanding's turtles utilize small wetlands compared to younger individuals. In addition, to explore how fast the traits of older females could increase in the population, we compared life tables based on traits of older turtles to a previously published life table for a stable population (Congdon et al. 1993).

An Overview of the ESGR Turtle Studies

The Study

In addition to the Blanding's turtles *(Emydoidea blandingii)*, 6,421 midland painted turtles *(Chrysemys picta marginata)* and 2,508 common snapping turtles *(Chelydra serpentina)* have been marked during the long-term study on the ESGR. Owen Sexton marked 92 Blanding's turtles between 1953–1957 (Sexton 1995) and from 1968–1973 Henry Wilbur marked 60 additional Blanding's turtles on the ESGR. During the current study (1975–2001), approximately 5,755 recaptures were made of 1,435 marked Blanding's turtles (350 adults, 200 juveniles, and 885 hatchlings), 817 X-radiographs of gravid females were taken, and 507 nests were observed. An additional 130 Blanding's turtles were marked during periodical searches of wetlands adjacent to the ESGR.

Study Site

Access to the ESGR is controlled by a 4-m high chain-link fence and locked gates; security of the s 615-ha research area has been a primary requirement for the success of the study. The ESGR is administered by the Museum of Zoology and is located in southeastern Michigan about 6 km west of the town of Pinckney in Livingston County (approximately 42°28'N, 84°00'W).

Aquatic areas on the ESGR (Fig. 1) include a 7.3-ha complex consisting of Southwest Swamp, Fishhook Marsh, and Crane Pond (Southwest Population), and a 5-ha complex consisting of East Marsh and Cattail Marsh (Southeast Population). Other aquatic areas include George and Burt Ponds (0.6 ha), Hidden Lake (0.4 ha), and Southeast Marsh (0.4 ha), and the Canal, Big Swamp and many small pot holes, wooded ponds, and temporary wetlands (Fig. 1). When combined, these smaller wetlands represent a substantial area of important habitats but are not considered permanent residences of turtles (Fig. 1).

Capture Methods

Turtles were captured in aquatic areas with baited hoop nets, fyke nets, basking traps, and by dip netting, muddling, or seining. They were also captured while at drift fences and on land moving between aquatic habitats or nesting sites. Each year from 1975–1986 and from 1991–1994 intensive aquatic trapping was carried out from early May through early September. Drift fences were usually monitored from April through June and during September and October. In addition, during all nesting seasons (mid-May to the beginning of July) from 1976–2001 four to seven people walked fences and searched nesting areas between 0600 h and 2300 h each day (for more details on research methods, see Congdon et al. 1983, 2000).

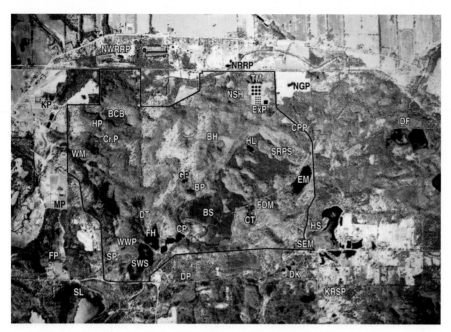

Fig. 1. Aquatic habitats and upland areas on the E. S. George Reserve. Wetlands commonly used as resident habitat by Blanding's turtles are labeled. Circular features and associated upland areas in northwest corner represent an enclosed experimental area. BCB (Big Cassandra Bog), BH (Buck Hollow), BP (Burt Pond), BS (Big Swamp), CrP (Cresent Pond), CP (Crane Pond), DF (Dragon Fly), DK (Doyle Kelly), DP (Doyle Pond), DT (Dollar Tamarack), EM (East Marsh), ExP (Experimental Ponds), FDM (Fox Den Marsh), FH (Fishhook Marsh), FP (Flare Pond), GP (George Pond), HL (Hidden Lake), HP (Hourglass Pond), HS (Horse Shoe), KP (Kaiser Ponds), KRSP (Kelly Road Spring Pool), MP (Maco Pond), NGP (North Gate Pond), NSH (North Sink Holes), NRRP (North Railroad Ponds), NWRRP (Northwestern Railroad Ponds), SL (Sayles Lake), SRPS (Stone Ring Ponds), SEM (Southeast Marsh), SP (Spring Pools); SWS (Southwest Swamp), TM (Tinkles Marsh), WM (West Marsh), WWP (West Woods Pond)

All juvenile and adult turtles were individually marked by notching or drilling the margins of the carapace. Prior to 1983, hatchlings were also individually marked, and from 1983 to 1992 all hatchling turtles from each nest were given identical nest cohort marks that were subsequently changed to unique individual marks when an individual was recaptured. The straight line lengths of both the plastron and carapace were measured at each capture. All turtles were then released at the point of capture or into water nearest their point of capture.

An Overview of Blanding's Turtle

The present range of Blanding's turtle (*Emydoidea blandingii*; family Emydidae) is restricted to south-central and southeastern Canada and north-central and the northeastern United States. Across their range, Blanding's turtles are similar in size with the exception of one large-bodied population in north-central Minnesota (Sajwaj 1998). Adults of both sexes are similar in body size and weight (Graham and Doyle 1977; Congdon and van Loben Sels 1991; Rowe 1992; Germano et al. 2000; Pappas et al. 2000). Female Blanding's turtles do not become sexually mature until they are at least 14 years old (Congdon and van Loben Sels 1993; Pappas et al. 2000). They produce a maximum of one clutch of eggs per year and some adult females do not reproduce every year (Congdon et al. 1983). Clutch Size ranges from 2 to 20 eggs with a mean of approximately 10 eggs (Congdon and van Loben Sels 1991; Congdon et al. 1983; Depari et al. 1987; Gibbons 1968; Graham and Doyle 1979; Pappas et al. 2000), and clutch size increases significantly with female body size (Congdon and van Loben Sels 1991; MacCulloch and Weller 1988; Pappas et al. 2000). Over 23 years of study on the ESGR, predation rates of nests was high ($\bar{x}$ = 78 %) but variable (minimum = 40 %, maximum = 100 %; Congdon et al. 2000). Among the nests that survived predation, 19.5 % failed entirely and, among the other surviving nests, 45 % had at least one egg fail (Congdon et al. 2000). Adult survivorship is high and some adults reach ages in excess of 70 years (Brecke and Moriarty 1989; Congdon and van Loben Sels 1991, 1993; Congdon et al. 1983, 2001). The traits of Blanding's turtles on the ESGR are summarized in Table 1. In southeastern Michigan hatchlings emerge from nests about 80 days after egg laying (mid-August–early October). Hatchling emergence occurs in one day for approximately half of the nests and over 2–4 days in the other half (Congdon et al. 1983).

Table 1. Traits of Blanding's turtles on the E. S. George Reserve based on data through the 2001 field season

Traits	Minimum	Maximum	Mean	N
Egg width (mm)	18.4	25.4	23.3	33
Egg mass (g)	5.4	14.9	12.0	27
Hatchling CL (mm)	26.0	39.0	35.0	872
Hatchling mass (g)	5.0	13.0	9.1	846
Female CL (mm)	161	215	186.9	208
Female body mass (g)	745	1432	1022.6	169
Age at maturity (yr)	14	21	17.7	27
Clutch size (#)	2	19	10.0	759
Reproductive rate (clutches/yr)	0	1	0.8	
Adult sex ratio (M/F)	–	–	1/3.8	
Male CL (mm)	161	231	192.3	62
Male body mass (g)	763	1488	1036.7	48

Aging in Blanding's Turtles

Indeterminate Growth

Adults of some turtle species continue to grow over their entire lifetimes, albeit at reduced rates compared to the growth rates of juveniles. Since reproductive output of adult turtles is almost always correlated with body size of adults (Congdon and Gibbons 1985), indeterminate growth is a relatively direct mechanism that results in increasing reproductive output of older turtles.

In contrast to turtles that exhibit indeterminate growth, adult Blanding's turtles increase in body size only for a few years after reaching sexual maturity (Congdon and van Loben Sels 1991; Pappas et al. 2000), with growth ceasing for both females and males a few years after reaching sexual maturity (Fig. 2 a, b). Female Blanding's turtles on the ESGR reach maturity between the ages of 14

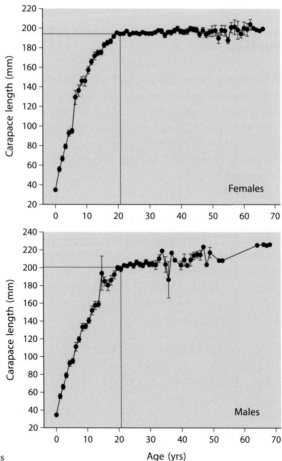

Fig. 2. Age-specific body sizes of male and female Blanding's turtles

and 21 years (Congdon and van Loben Sels 1993) and have a potential repro-ductive lifespan of over 55 years (Brecke and Moriarty 1989; Congdon et al. 2001; Pappas et al. 2000). Variation in growth rates among juveniles combined with variation in ages at sexual maturity results in the major source of variation in body sizes among adult females (Congdon and van Loben Sels 1991, 1993). Indeterminate growth, therefore, is not a major mechanism for the evolution of longevity in the ESGR population of Blanding's turtles.

Almost a decade after Congdon and van Loben Sels (1993) examined the ESGR Blanding's turtles for evidence of reproductive senescence, Congdon et al. (2001) tested predictions from the Relative Reproductive Rate and Senescence hypotheses by comparing reproductive parameters and adult survivorships of three age groups of female Blanding's turtles. At the end of a 20-year study period, maximum ages of females within the young and middle age groups were 39 and 48 years old, respectively. Females in the oldest age group were assigned minimum ages based on their capture as adults between 1953–1957; at the end of the study period the turtles were all greater than 66 years old.

Traits not Supporting the Senescence or Relative Reproductive Rate Hypotheses (Table 2)

As expected, based on the lack of indeterminate growth in Blanding's adults, body size was not larger in older age groups and, therefore, did not influence differences in reproductive output of the age groups. Sizes of eggs and hatch-lings were not different among age groups, indicating that, in the absence of body size effects, parental investment (allocation to individual neonates) is not influenced by age. The number of hatchlings produced per nest was also similar among age groups.

Table 2. Traits of Blanding's turtles that support the Relative Reproductive Rate hypoth-esis, the Senescence hypothe-sis, or neither hypothesis of aging

Hypotheses	Traits
Relative Reproductive Rate	Clutch size
	Reproductive frequency
	Adult survivorship
	Nest predation rate
Senescence	Embryo development
	Nest success
Neither	Indeterminate growth
	Body size
	Egg size
	Hatchling size
	# Hatchlings per nest

Traits that Supported the Senescence Hypotheses (Table 2)

The proportion of nests that survived predation but then failed entirely due to developmental problems was lowest in the young age group and increased with age among groups. As a result, nest success was highest in younger turtles.

Traits that Supported the Relative Reproductive Rate Hypotheses (Table 2)

Once the small differences in body size were adjusted among individuals, females in the oldest age group had the largest average clutch size and the lowest nest predation rates. Whereas recapture frequencies of females were similar for all age groups, reproductive frequency was highest in the oldest age group, and similar between the young and middle age groups. Over the same 20-year period, survivorship of females in the oldest age group was significantly higher than that of the middle age group. Survivorship of the youngest turtles was not compared because not all of them were captured early enough to be present as adults over the entire 20-year period.

Trait Comparisons that May be Sample Biased

Three of the traits (nest predation rates, embryo mortality, and nest success) compared among age groups had the potential to be biased by sampling methods. Because data on nests were collected from many nesting areas over 24 years, among-group differences in the distribution of nests over time and space could have biased some results. Stronger evidence for age-specific differences in nest success due to embryo survival will require common garden experiments where environmental differences are controlled. In addition, since the numbers of hatchlings produced per nest were similar among age groups, support or lack thereof should be viewed with caution.

Conclusions from Tests of Aging Hypotheses

The major cause of variation in body size among adult Blanding's turtles was not indeterminate growth; therefore, changes in reproductive characteristics that are positively associated with body size of female Blanding's turtles are not related to age of adults (Congdon and van Loben Sels 1991; Congdon et al. 2001).

Overall, the comparison of traits among the age groups provides the strongest support for the Relative Reproductive Rate hypothesis (Table 2). Increased reproductive output of older Blanding's turtle females results from increases in clutch size, reproductive frequency, and adult survivorship in the oldest age group compared to younger age groups. The fact that traits promoting increases in the proportion of late versus early births remain detectable in the oldest Blanding's turtles females in the population, does not support the assertion that ". . . senescence always creeps in" (Hamilton 1966).

Male Reproductive Success

From 1997–2000, blood samples were taken of all adult males and females captured on the ESGR (and three from immediately adjacent areas). In addition, 30 nests (239 hatchlings) with known mothers (observed constructing nests) and four nests (27 hatchlings) with unknown mothers were collected on the ESGR and tail tips were taken for genetic analyses. All adults and hatchlings from the population were genotyped at 10 microsatellite loci (for methodology, see Osentoski 2001) and fathers were assigned to hatchlings using the likelihood approach (Marshall et al. 1998). Male reproductive success was defined as the number of hatchlings assigned to a given male over the four-year period. The percentage of males genotyped was estimated at 95 % of the total population (51 males) over the 20 years of study (Congdon and Gibbons 1996).

Of the 266 hatchlings genotyped, 103 (38.7 %) were assigned to males from the ESGR. Examination of capture histories suggested the percentage of unassigned hatchlings was related to females nesting on the ESGR that had mated with unmarked males that did not reside on the ESGR (Osentoski 2001). Analyses of all ESGR males sampled indicated that reproductive success was nonrandomly distributed among individuals (Fig. 3). Male reproductive success differed significantly from a Poisson distribution ($X^2_{5, 0.05} = 151.4$, $p < 0.001$), with more males than expected siring greater than four offspring and more males than expected siring zero offspring (21 males, 39 %).

When examined separately, both male age and body size contributed significantly to explaining the variance in male reproductive success; however, when examined simultaneously only age explained a significant portion of the variance (Table 3). Aggressive male-male interaction (Kinney 1999; Rowe and Moll 1977) could explain some of the success of larger male Blanding's turtles but, as

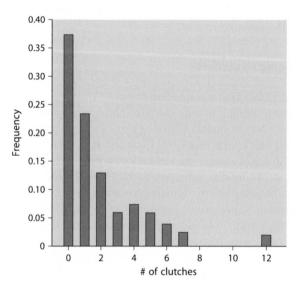

Fig. 3. Distribution of reproductive success of males on the E. S. George reserve. Distribution is significantly different from Poisson ($X^2_{5, 0.05} = 151.4$, $p < 0.001$)

Table 3. Results of a general linear model using the Poisson family of response distributions with male reproductive success as the dependent variable[a]

Independent variable	DF	estimate	Standard error	z-value	p-value
(Intercept)		−2.6438	0.9631	−2.745	0.006
Body size (ALL males)	51	0.0191	0.0047	4.047	.00005
(Intercept)		−2.4338	1.0484	−2.322	0.020
Body size[a]	39	0.0182	0.0051	3.519	0.0004[a]
(Intercept)		0.2835	0.2445	1.160	0.246
AGE[a]	39	0.0303	0.0074	4.109	0.00003[a]
(Intercept)		−1.2775	1.1540	−1.107	0.2683
Body size[a]	39	0.0089	0.0064	1.389	0.1647
AGE[a]	39	0.0224	0.0091	2.451	0.0143[a]

[a] Only males that could be accurately aged were included in the analyses

noted for females, indeterminate growth of adults does not contribute much to variation in adult body size.

Use of small wetlands by Blanding's turtles

Although large, permanent marshes and swamps are typically resident wetlands of Blanding's turtles (Fig. 4 a), data from several sources indicate that small (< 4.0 ha) wetlands are important to adults as sources of ephemeral, but concentrated food sources (e.g., amphibian and insect larvae), for mating, and refugia during nesting migrations by females and during hatchling dispersal from nests (Pappas et al. 2000; Piepgras and Lang 2000; Kinney 1999; Ross and Anderson 1990; Butler and Graham 1995; this study Fig. 4 a, b). Small wetlands used by Blanding's turtles on the ESGR include many types ranging from clear, permanent, spring-fed wooded pools to shallow, ephemeral, duckweed-covered swamps. Individual turtles may visit small wetlands more than 1-km from their resident marsh, and at least some individuals appear to make similar movements among wetlands over a number of years.

Movements of adult turtles among wetlands in early spring, combined with observations of courtship in March and April, suggest that spring is a peak mating period (Graham and Doyle 1979; Baker and Gillingham 1983; Herman et al. 1995; Sajwaj 1998; Joyal et al. 2000; Pappas et al. 2000; Piepgras and Lang 2000; ESGR studies). However, Blanding's turtles have been observed mating in all months of their activity season, and a second peak in breeding activity may also occur in the fall (Graham and Doyle 1977; Kinney 1999; Pappas et al. 2000; Piepgras and Lang 2000). Movements among wetlands by males may increase the probability of males mating with more females (Morreale et al. 1984). Females visit small wetlands located near nesting areas to rehydrate (Kiviat 1997; Kinney et al. 1998; Congdon et al. 2000) before and after strenuous activities such as nesting migrations, nest construction, egg laying, and covering the nest. Newly emerged hatchlings in the fall also use small wetlands near nesting

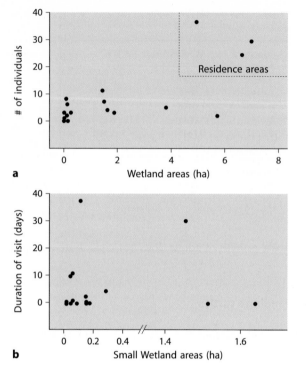

Fig. 4. Relationship between wetland area and (a) number of individuals captured and (b) duration of visits during the 1997 and 1998 field seasons

areas for temporary refugia (Butler and Graham 1995) and probably also to hydrate. The ability of hatchlings to find and utilize small wetlands may substantially contribute to their survival during what is presumed to be a particularly vulnerable period (Ehrenfeld 1979).

Blanding's turtle is primarily carnivorous (Cahn 1937; Lagler 1943; Penn 1950; Graham and Doyle 1977; Kofron and Schreiber 1985; Ross 1989) and feeds on seasonally abundant tadpoles and larval salamanders. Small isolated wetlands are apparently utilized by both sexes as sites for harvesting ephemeral resources (e.g., amphibian and insect larvae). Radiotelemetry studies combined with mark recapture data on the ESGR indicate that, during mid-summer, both male and female turtles sometimes remain in small wetlands for periods exceeding 60 days (Fig. 4 b). Three such small wetlands (Spring Pools, Stone Ring Pool, Badlands Pool) are relatively permanent, spring-fed shrub swamps that contain high densities of larval amphibians (e.g., *Rana sylvatica* and *Ambystoma* spp.). However, since courtship and mating have been observed in small wetlands (Kinney 1999; Pappas et al. 2000), males may benefit from increased resources and mating opportunities. If the experience of older individuals of both sexes results in improved abilities in using ephemeral wetlands (e.g., initially finding them, reduced effort to return to them, and knowing when to visit them), they should have increased benefits and reduced costs and risks associated with their use of them. In addition, enhanced use of small wetlands by older adults of both sexes may result in a higher probability of matings between old individuals.

General Conclusions

Our review of the life history and aging of Blanding's turtles summarizes what is known about the population on the University of Michigan's E. S. George Reserve in general and compares younger females to a group of females marked as adults between 1953 and 1957 (Sexton 1995). The oldest group of females had higher survivorships, reproduced more frequently, and had larger clutch sizes than did younger females. In addition, a preliminary genetic analysis indicated that older males had higher reproductive success than did younger males. We developed an age-based scenario of differential use of temporary wetlands as a mechanism supporting the larger allocation to reproduction by old females. The scenario would also place old males in the proximity of old females during periods of high resources and intense breeding activity.

Using life table analyses, we compared cohorts of the oldest Blanding's turtles (with traits of increased fecundity and survivorship) to a cohort of females with traits that result in a stable population (Congdon et al. 1993) to explore how fast cohorts of old females could double in numbers within the population (Fig. 5). Increasing annual fecundity by 0.5 and 1.0 eggs for old females resulted in population doubling times of 793 and 444 years, respectively, whereas increasing adult survivorship by 0.02 resulted in a population doubling time of 226 years, or half the time to double the population that occurred by increasing fecundity by one egg. Increasing both fecundity by 1.0 egg and survivorship by

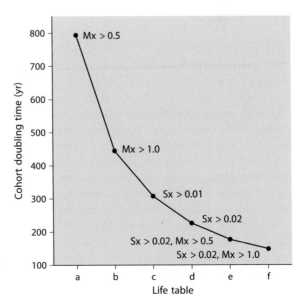

Fig. 5. Changes in doubling time for a cohort of *Emydoidea blandingii* females that allow increased Mx (fecundity) and Sx (survivorship of adults) in individuals age 50 years or older compared to a life table for a stable population (Congdon et al. 1993; females mature between 14 and 21 years, embryo, average annual juvenile (ages 1–13) and adult survivorships of 0.26, 0.78 and 0.96, respectively, and Mx (annual fecundity) of four female producing eggs. All life table calculations hold other variables constant, while increasing 1) Mx by 0.1 eggs, and 2) Sx (survivorship) of adults to increase by 0.02 in females older than 49 yrs of age

0.02 (representing the reproductive output and survivorship of the oldest age group in the ESGR population; Congdon et al. 2001) reduced the doubling time of 148 years (Fig. 5).

Assuming that there is a genetic component to attainment of old age by Blanding's turtles, then selection for longevity (represented by the doubling times resulting from the above cohort comparisons) could be driven to some extent by increased ability to find and more efficiently use temporary wetlands. Efficient use of wetlands by older individuals (compared to younger individuals) could support the increased production of offspring by older females and the increased probability of matings between old males and females (i.e., resulting offspring would have two sets of "old genes").

The distinctive suite of life history characteristics coupled with their protective shell appears to promote overall and reproductive longevity of turtles. Intensive long-term studies of turtles (Stickel 1950; Legler 1960; Galbraith et al. 1989; Gibbons 1990; Congdon and Gibbons 1996; Iverson and Smith 1993; van Loben Sels et al. 1997; Pappas et al. 2000) have focused primarily on the difficult task of describing the ecology and life histories of species' populations. Long-term observations of individuals have provided information on longevity that goes well beyond the survivorship of captive or exceptional individuals. Rather, the observations have provided age structures and probabilities of survivorship for individuals of different ages. Growing appreciation of current issues related to the biology of aging can further focus efforts of individuals conducting long-term studies on obtaining data on the oldest-aged individuals in the population; such a focus can provide new and contrasting views of aging (Congdon et al. 2001).

Acknowledgments

We thank the Foundation IPSEN for awarding the senior author the "Longevity Prix" based on the long-term study of turtles. We appreciate the University of Michigan and its Museum of Zoology for administering and maintaining the E. S. George Reserve as a world class research area. J. Whitfield Gibbons has provided continued and enthusiastic support of the study. The following people made notable contributions to the study: Sue and Harold Avery, Margaret Burkman, Carl and Melvin Congdon, Scott Connelly, Nancy, Barbara, and Bob Dickson, Ruth Estes, Rose Fama, Robert Fischer, Matthew Hinz, Mark Hutcheson, Joyce Klevering, Tal Novak, Todd Quinter, Willem Roosenburg, Todd Sajwaj. Earlier drafts of this manuscript were improved by comments from Ronald Brooks, Nancy Dickson, Whit Gibbons, and William Hopkins. Funding was provided by NSF Grants DEB-74-070631, DEB-79-06301, BSR-84-00861 and BSR-90-19771. Our research was also supported by Financial Assistance Award Number DE-FC09-96SR18546, from the United States Department of Energy to the University of Georgia Research Foundation.

References

Baker RE, Gillingham JC (1983) An analysis of courtship behavior in Blanding's turtles, *Emydoidea blandingii*. Herpetologica 39: 166–173.

Barwick RE (1982) The growth and ecology of the gecko *Hoplodactylus duvauceli* at Brothers Islands. In: Neman DG (ed.) New Zealand herpetology. Wildlife Service, Wellington, 377–391.

Bodie R, Semlitsch RC (2000) Size-specific mortality and natural selection in freshwater turtles. Copeia 2000: 732–739.

Brecke BJ, Moriarty JJ (1989) *Emydoidea blandingii* (Blanding's Turtle) longevity. Herpetol Rev 20 (2): 53.

Butler BO, Graham TE (1995) Early post-emergent behavior and habitat selection in hatchling Blanding's turtles *(Emydoidea blandingii)*, in Massachusetts. Chelonian Conserv Biol. 1: 187–196.

Cagle FR (1944) Sexual maturity in the female of the turtle *Pseudemys scripta elegans*. Copeia 1944: 149–152.

Cahn AR (1937) The turtles of Illinois. Illinois Biological Monogrphs. Vol. 35.

Charlesworth B (1995) Evolution in age-structured populations, Chicago, University of Chicago Press.

Cole LC (1954) The population consequences of life history phenomena. Quart Rev Biol. 29: 103–137.

Congdon JD, Gibbons JW (1985) Egg components and reproductive characteristics of turtles: relationships to body size. Herpetologica 41: 194–205.

Congdon JD, Gibbons JW (1990) The evolution of turtle life histories. In: JW Gibbons (ed) Life history and ecology of the Slider turtle Washington DC, Smithsonian Institution Press: 45–54.

Congdon JD, Gibbons JW (1996) Structure and dynamics of a turtle community over two decades. In: Cody MC, Smallwood San Diego. (eds). Long-term studies of vertebrate communities. Academic Press, Inc. 137–159.

Congdon JD, van Loben Sels RC (1991) Growth and body size in the Blanding's turtles *(Emydoidea blandingii)*: relationships to reproduction. Can J Zool 69: 239–245.

Congdon JD, van Loben Sels RC (1993) Reproductive characteristics and body size: relationships with attainment of sexual maturity and age in Blanding's turtles *(Emydoidea blandingii)*. J Evol Biol 6: 547–557.

Congdon JD, Tinkle DW, Breitenbach GL, van Loben Sels RC (1983) Nesting ecology and hatching success in the turtle *Emydoidea blandingii*. Herpetologic 39: 417–429.

Congdon JD, Dunham AE, van Loben Sels RC (1993) Delayed sexual maturity and demographics of Blanding's turtles *(Emydoidea blandingii)*: implications for conservation and management of long-lived organisms. J Conserv Biol 7: 826–833.

Congdon JD, Nagle RD, Dunham AE, Beck C, Kinney OM, Yeomans SR (1999) An experimental analysis of the relationship between body size and survivorship of hatchling snapping turtles *(Chelydra serpentina)*: an evaluation of the "bigger is better" hypothesis. Oecologia 121: 224–235.

Congdon JD, Nagle RD, Kinney OM, Osentoski M, Avery H, van Loben Sels RC, Tinkle DW (2000) Nesting ecology, and embryo mortality: implications for the demography of Blanding's turtles *(Emydoidea blandingii)*. Chelonian Conserv Biol 3: 569–579.

Congdon JD, Nagle RA, Kinney OM, van Loben Sels RC (2001) Hypotheses of aging in a long-lived vertebrate (Blanding's turtle, *Emydoidea blandingii*). Exp Gerontol 36: 813–827.

Dunham AE, Overall KL, Porter WP (1989) Implications of ecological energetics and biophysical and developmental constraints for life-history variation in dinosaurs. Geol Soc Amer Special Paper 238.

Ehrenfeld DW (1979) Behavior associated with nesting. In: Harless M, Morlock H (eds.) Turtles: perspectives and research. John Wiley and Sons, New York, 417–434.

Finch CE (1999) Longevity without aging: possible examples. In: Robine JM, Forette B, Franceschi C, Allard M (eds) The paradoxes of longevity. Springer Verlag, Paris 1–10.

Fox SF (1978) Natural selection on behavioral phenotypes of the lizard, *Uta stansburiana*. Ecology 59: 834–847.

Galbraith DA, Brooks RJ, Obbard ME (1989) The influence of growth rate on age and body size at maturity in female snapping turtles *(Chelydra serpentina)*. Copeia 1989: 896–904.

Germano DJ, Bury RB, Jennings M (2000) Growth and population structure of *Emydoidea blandingii* from western Nebraska. Chelonian Conserv Biol 3: 618–625.

Gibbons JW (1968) Observations on the ecology and population dynamics of the Blanding's turtle, *Emydoidea blandingii*. Can J Zool 46: 288–290.

Gibbons JW (1969) Ecology and population dynamics of the chicken turtle, *Deirochelys reticularia*. Copeia 1969: 669–676.

Gibbons JW (1976) Aging phenomena in reptiles. In: Elias MF, Eleftheriou BE, Elias PK (eds) Experimental aging research. EAR Inc., Bar Harbor, ME USA, 454–475.

Graham TE, Doyle TS (1977) Growth and population characteristics of Blanding's turtles, *Emydoidea blandingii* in Massachusetts. Herpetologica 33: 410–414.

Graham TE, Doyle TS (1979) Dimorphism, courtship, eggs and hatchlings of the Blanding's turtle, *Emydoidea blandingii* (Reptilia, Testudinies, Emydidae) in Massachusetts. J Herpetol 13: 125–127.

Hamilton WD (1966) The moulding of senescence by natural selection. J Theoret Biol 12: 12–45.

Herman TB, Power TD, Eaton BR (1995) Population status of Blanding's turtles *(Emydoidea blandingii)* in Nova Scotia. Can Field Naturalist 109: 182–191.

Iverson J, Smith GR (1993) Reproductive ecology of the painted turtle *(Chrysemys picta)* in the Nebraska Sandhills. Copeia 1993 (1): 1–21.

Janzen FJ, Tucker JK, Paukstis GL (2000) Experimental analysis of an early life-history stage: selection on size of hatchling turtles. Ecology 81: 2290–2304.

Joyal LA, McColloough M, Hunter Jr, ML (2000) Population structure and reproductive ecolog of Blanding's turtle *(Emydoidea blandingii)* in Maine, near the northeastern edge of its range. Chelonian Conserv Biol 3: 580–588.

Kinney OM (1999) Movements and habitat use of Blanding's turtles in southeast Michigan: implications for conservation and management. M. S. thesis. University of Georgia.

Kinney OM, Nagle RD, Congdon JD (1998) Water transport by nesting painted turtles *(Chrysemys picta marginata)* in Michigan. Chelonian Conserv Biol 3: 71–76.

Kirkwood T (1999) Time of Our Lives. Oxford University Press, New York.

Kiviat E (1997) Blanding's turtle habitat requirements and implications for conservation in Dutchess County, New York. Proceedings: Conservation, restoration, and management of tortoises and turtles – an international conference. New York Turtle and Tortoise Society, New York, 377–382.

Kofron CP, Schrieber AA (1985) Ecology of two endangered aquatic turtles in Missouri: Kinosternon flavescens and *Emydoidea blandingii*. J Herpetol 19: 27–40.

Lagler KF (1943) Food habits and economic relations of the turtles of Michigan with special reference to fish management. Am Midland Naturalist 29: 257–312.

Legler JM (1960) Natural history of the ornate box turtle, Terrapene ornata ornata Agassiz. Univ. Kansas Publication of the Museum of Natural History, Vol 11: 527–669.

MacCulloch RD, Weller WF (1988) Some aspects of reproduction in a Lake Erie population of Blanding's turtle, *Emydoidea blandingii*. Can J Zool 66: 2317–2319.

Marshall TC, Slate J, Kruuk LEB, Pemberton JM (1998). Statistical confidence for likelihood-based paternity inference in natural populations. Mol Ecol 7: 639–655.

Medawar PB (1952) An unsolved problem of biology. HK Lewis, London.

Moll EO (1979) Reproductive cycles and adaptations. In: Harless M, Morlock H (eds) Turtles: perspectives and research. John Wiley and Sons, New York, 305–331.

Morreale SJ, Gibbons JW, Congdon JD (1984) Significance of activity and movement in the yellow-bellied slider turtle *(Pseudemys scripta)*. Can J Zool 62: 1038–1042.

Osentoski MF (2001) Population genetic structure and male reproductive success of a Blanding's turtle *(Emydoidea blandingii)* population in southeastern Michigan. Doctoral Dissertation, University of Miami (FL).

Pappas MJ, Brecke BJ, Congdon JD (2000) The Blanding's turtle of Weaver Dunes, Minnesota. Chelonian Conserv Biol 3: 557–568.

Penn GH (1950) Utilization of crawfishes by cold-blooded vertebrates in the eastern United States. Am Midland Naturalist 44: 643–658.

Piepgras SJ, Lang JW (2000) Spatial ecology of Blanding's turtle in central Minnesota. Chelonian Conserv Biol 3: 589.

Rose MR (1996) Towards an evolutionary demography. In: Rose MR, Lauder GV (eds) Adaptation. San Diego: Academic Press, 96–107.

Ross DA (1989) Population ecology of painted and Blanding's turtles *(Chrysemys picta* and *Emydoidea blandingii)* in central Wisconson. Transact Wisc Acad Sci Art let Wisc Acad Sci 77: 77–84.

Ross DA, Anderson RK (1990) Habitat use, movements, and nesting of *Emydoidea blandingii* in central Wisconsin. J Herpetol 24: 6–12.

Rowe JW (1992) Observations of body size, growth, and reproduction in Blanding's turtles *(Emydoidea blandingii)* from western Nebraska. Can J Zool 70: 1690–1695.

Sajwaj TD (1998) Seasonal and daily patterns of body temperature and thermal behavior in a central Minnesota population of Blanding's turtles *(Emydoidea blandingii)*. MS Thesis, University of North Dakota, Grand Forks, ND.

Sexton OJ (1995) Miscellaneous comments on the natural history of Blanding's turtle *(Emydoidea blandingii)*. Trans Missouri Acad Sci 29: 1–13.

Sinervo B, Doughty P, Huey RB, Zamudio K (1992) Allometric engineering: a causal analysis of natural selection on offspring size. Science 258: 1927–1930.

Stickel LF (1950) Populations and home range relationships of the box turtle, Terrapene carolina (Linnaeus). Ecol Mono 20: 351–378.

van Loben Sels RC, Congdon JD, Austin JT (1997) Life history and ecology of the Sonoran mud turtle *(Kinosternon sonoriense)* in southeast Arizona: a preliminary report. Chelonian Conserv Biol 2: 338–344.

Wilbur HM, Morin PJ (1988) Life history evolution in turtles. In: Gans C, Huey R (eds) Biology of the reptilia Vol. 16 b. Alan R. Liss, Inc., New York, 396–447.

Williams GC (1957) Pleiotropy, natural selection, and the evolution of senescence. Evolution 11: 398–411.

Williams GC (1966) Adaptation and natural selection: a critique of some current evolutionary thought. Princeton University Press, Princeton, New Jersey.

Lipoprotein Genes and Diet in the Evolution of Human Intelligence and Longevity

C. E. Finch and C. B. Stanford

Summary

Humans have evolved two traits that differ from other great apes and that appear to be antagonistic: slower aging despite a major increase in meat eating. The three great apes – chimpanzees, gorillas, and orangutans – and the gibbons do not live more than 60 years under the best circumstances. The longevity of humans evolved despite the higher exposure to cholesterol and other fats than in other great apes. Laboratory chimpanzees are highly sensitive to dietary fat, which causes hyperlipidemia, accelerated vascular disease, and rapid increases in myocardial infarcts. Furthermore, clinical and animal studies indicate that blood cholesterol is a risk factor in Alzheimer Disease. We conclude that the evolution of "meat-adaptive genes" was crucial to the evolution of human longevity.

The hominoid lineage has been mainly vegetarian for more than 25 million years, according to evidence from dentition and the current diet of great apes. The gorilla and bonobo feed almost exclusively on fruit, leaves, and nuts. The chimpanzee is a partial exception, because some individuals hunt and eat other small mammals. However, other individuals, as well as neighboring groups, may not eat meat.

During the past several million years, meat eating increased progressively, more – or less in concert with increases of brain size, longer postnatal care, and increasingly sophisticated tool manufacture and hunting strategies. Stone-age hunters clearly targeted brains and bone marrow, which provide year-around sources of fat that are used to metabolize protein. Limitations on dietary fat or carbohydrate restrict the amount of muscle that can be eaten without inducing ammonia toxicity because of the ceiling on urea production. Humans are clearly adapted to consume much more meat for energy than, for example, chimpanzees, which forage in 90 % smaller areas than present hunter-gatherers. The increased life expectancy is of particular importance to those aged 20–50, when most human hunter-gatherers are their most productive.

The increase of dietary fat would be expected to select for meat-adaptive genes that reduce hyperlipidemia with associated risks to heart and brain. A rapidly emerging literature is consistent in the ability of elevated cellular cholesterol to increase production of the amyloid β-peptide. There are also indications that elevated neuronal cholesterol is associated with NFT formation, particularly in Nieman-Pick disease, a cholesterol storage disorder.

Finch et al. (Eds.)
Brain and Longevity
© Springer-Verlag Berlin Heidelberg 2003

The apoE allele system could be important, because primates have only the E4 allele, which promotes higher blood cholesterol and increased risk of vascular disease and AD. The apoE4 isoform is relatively vulnerable to cleavage into a fragment that causes tau-hyperphosphorylation. Other genes may increase host resistance to infectious agents in uncooked organs (viruses and prions found in marrow and brain; enteric parasites). Muscle is also rich in metals (heme-iron, copper and zinc), which would involve genes of detoxification.

It is clear that the evolution of meat-adaptive genes was required for human longevity. These adaptations also pose questions about the applicability of caloric restriction to health and aging in normal humans, i.e., those without obesity who exercise. More generally, some racial groups show different incidence of AD between national populations, which may involve the degree of vegetarianism. Thus, pursuit of evolutionary questions may also give important insights into human risk factors.

Introduction

Humans have large brains, prolonged postnatal development and increased adult life spans by comparison with their closest relatives: bonobos, chimpanzees, gorillas, and orangutans. During evolution, humans also made a major shift in diet from the primarily vegetarian diets of the anthropoid clade to the major consumption of mammalian organs by paleolithic humans. Here we consider the consequences to health of the increased meat diet. We argue that this diet shift selected for particular categories of genes that modulate cholesterol, metals, and infectious agents, which we designate as "meat adaptive genes". Apolipoprotein E (apoE) in particular is a candidate for an important role in these transitions that allow major increases in life span, despite the dangers of meat eating. Chimpanzees that hunt and consume small mammals may have pioneered this trend.

Aging in Chimpanzees

Evidence for Geriatric Chimpanzees

Sixty years is the maximum life span reported for captive and wild populations of chimpanzee, bonobo, gorilla, and orangutan (Hill et al. 2001; Kaplan et al. 2000; Nowak and Paradiso 1983). The life expectancy of adult chimpanzees is < 50 % of humans (Table 1) (Kaplan et al. 2000; Hill et al. 2001). As another index of faster aging, chimpanzees show markedly earlier acceleration of mortality rates during aging in feral populations (Hill et al. 2001). Mortality rate acceleration is widely used as a demographic marker of senescence (Finch et al. 1990; Finch 1990; Vaupel et al. 1998). By the age of 35–40 years, zoo and natural populations show strong accelerations of mortality rates, which is about

Table 1. The life expectancy of chimpanzees[a] and humans

	Life expectancy at birth	at 15 years	Survival (%) to 50 years	60 years	70 years	Maximum life span (years)
Wild chimpanzees Kibale, site of lowest mortality (Hill et al. 2001)	15 years	15 years	9	< 1	0	60 (also zoo)
Hunter-gatherers Aché, precontact; (Kaplan et al. 2000)	30 years	39 years	42	30	15	> 75
Modern industrial	> 75 years	> 65 years	95	90	70	>110

[a] Mortality of chimpanzees is very high in the first year (20 %) and can be even higher in zoos than in wild populations (Courtenay and Santow 1989; Kaplan et al. 2001). Thereafter and until age 15, zoo and wild population have similar demographics. At age 25, > 90 % of zoo animals survive five more years, which is about two-fold more than in the wild.

20 years earlier than in hunter-gatherers (Hill et al. 2001; Kaplan et al. 2000) and all other human populations (Finch 1990; Vaupel et al. 1998).

But do chimpanzees and other apes really age faster than humans would under primitive conditions, in correspondence with the earlier accelerations of mortality? Limited observations support this hypothesis, as surveyed below and in Table 2. Field workers speak of animals aged 35 as "old" (Hill et al. 2001). At Gombe, adults in their last years become increasingly frail and emaciated (Goodall 1983). As stated by Hill et al. (2001): "... *two very senile females believed to be* > 45 *years...*" (Wrangham) and "... *a white-haired and bent old male who lived another 13 years...* (Nishida); one male (the oldest at Kibale) was described as "past prime" and disappeared while still "looking strong".
This latter observation points out the difficulty in assessing vitality from external appearance. The wearing of teeth from chewing of abrasive materials may be a major source of disability, which by impairing food intake, could be a factor in emaciation and osteoporosis (Zihlman et al. 1989). In elephants, tooth wear is considered to be a major factor in frailty at later ages (Sikes 1971; see detailed discussion in Finch 1990, pp 197–199). The slower movements of older chimpanzees (Goodall 1986; Stanford, unpublished) suggest either, or both, neurological impairments of painful joints. Histological analysis of brain aging is discussed in the next section. Little is known about vision (e.g., lens opacity) or hearing in aging chimpanzees.

The causes of spontaneous death in the wild are unknown. In captive chimpanzees, case reports describe death from myocardial infarcts as early as eight years (adolescent female) (Manning 1942). Congestive heart failure in a 26-year-old male was associated with brain damage, which included "perivascular hemorrhage and... severe status spongiosis" of the brain (Hansen et al. 1984). Oral infections may also harbor bacteria that cause heart disease (see Table 2, foot-

Table 2. The geriatric profile of chimpanzees at Gombe[a]

Hill et al. (2001)	Young, 15–20 years	Old, > 35 years
Body mass		Emaciation before death is common
Hair	Thick	Thinning on shoulders, head, lower back
	Black	Browner and grayer
	Glossy	Less sheen (implies decreased sebaceous gland secretions or decreased grooming)
Movements	Vigorous	Slower
Sex differences		"Looked really old": Males 3 %, females 11 %
Skin (facial)	Light creases	Sagging and wrinkled
Teeth	Unworn	Worn
	Not broken	May be broken

[a] Tooth wear from vegetarian diets by limiting food intake could be a factor in frailty and emaciation of chimpanzees, as observed in many other species of herbivores in which a critical limit of tooth erosion is a regular outcome of aging (reviewed in Finch 1990, pp. 197–201). In deer, wearing of teeth to the gum with exposure of the pulp cavity is associated with increased infections (Severinghaus 1949). Moreover, periodontal disease can harbor bacteria that can enter the circulation to cause cardiovascular disease and endocarditis in humans (Bate et al. 2000; Mattila et al. 2000). For example, endocarditis and valvular fibrosis in a 12-years-old chimpanzee was attributed to chronic trench mouth by Schmidt (1978).

note). A thorough geriatric profile would be very informative, particularly with comparisons to wild and zoo chimpanzees, bonobos, and gorillas. According to zoo records for gorillas, cardiovascular disease (fibrosis) is a major cause of mortality (Lindsay and Chaikoff 1966; Schmidt 1978), with a high incidence of aortic dissection (T Meehan and L Munson, personal communication).

Brain Aging

Not much is known about brain aging in two of the four great ape species, the chimpanzee and the orangutan, which have similar maximum life spans of about 60 years. Only three old chimpanzee brains have been examined for neuropathology with immunohistochemistry (Gearing et al. 1994, 1996). The two oldest were females aged 56 (Bula) and 59 years (Gamma) from the Yerkes Primate Center. Both brains had distinct deposits of the amyloid β-peptide (Aβ) in the form of cerebrovascular amyloid and diffuse amyloid plaques in the cerebral cortex and hippocampus. These deposits were immunoreactive for apolipoprotein E (apoE), as found in Alzheimer disease (AD), but were much sparser than in human AD or in aging rhesus monkeys (Price et al. 1991). Moreover, the Aβ peptide composition differed. In human brains, cerebrovascular Aβ is mainly Aβ1–40 (40 amino acids long), whereas plaque amyloid is mainly Aβ1–42. Chimpanzee plaques had relatively more Aβ1–40 than human plaques, as judged by the 70 % larger ratios of Aβ1–40: Aβ1–42 shown by immunohisto-chemistry (Gearing et al. 1996). The additional two amino acids in Aβ1–42 cause its greater aggregation in biophysical studies and are associated with greater neurotoxicity (references in Klein et al. 2001).

However, in contrast to brains in human AD or in aging monkeys, the two oldest chimpanzee brains did not have any indication of degenerating neurites in these amyloid deposits. Neurofibrillary degeneration was absent and Alz-50 immunoreactivity for hyperphosphorylated tau, though present, was confined to rare neurons. This finding is important because neuritic or neurofibrillary degeneration, with highly aggregated and hyperphosphorylated tau in microtu-bules, is a major characteristic of AD. Neuritic degeneration with abnormal, hyperphosphorylated tau is found in many other primate brains during aging (Finch and Sapolsky 1999, Härtig et al. 2000), e.g., in the rhesus monkey brains that were included for comparison in the study by Gearing et al. (1996). The age progression of these changes in apes is not known. One male chimpanzee, aged 45 and terminally ill, had no cerebrovascular amyloid or diffuse amyloid plaques (S. Mirra, personal communication); he was only slightly younger than the two males that showed modest amyloid deposits and may not be representa-tive, in view of the findings of amyloid in younger orangutans, as discussed below.

Orangutans have similarly mild brain changes, as documented in a larger sample (N = 12). Sparse, diffuse amyloid deposits are observed by 21 years and may be more prevalent than in the two much older chimpanzees described above (Gearing et al. 1996, 1997; Selkoe et al. 1987). In individuals aged > 20 years, the amyloid was predominantly Aβ1–40 and colocalized with apoE in both plaques and vascular deposits, as in chimpanzees (Gearing et al. 1996, 1997). The oldest, at 46 years, showed modest numbers of plaques and vascular immunostaining with antisera to Aβ1–28, with a much lower prevalence than in the human AD or aged rhesus brains that were included as positive controls (Selkoe et al. 1987). No amyloid was found in a 10-year-old orangutan brain (Gearing et al. 1997), which would be expected for a primate in early adulthood. Also notable, the orangutan did not have obvious reactive glia (microglia, astro-cytes) in association with plaques (Gearing et al. 1997); in contrast, aging rhe-sus have reactive microglia around their senile plaques (Härtig et al. 1997), as well as abnormal neuronal processes (Price et al. 1991). Like the chimpanzees, these orangutans did not show evidence of neurofibrillary or neuritic degenera-tion (Gearing et al. 1996, 1997).

The absence of neurofibrillary changes and neuritic degeneration during aging in great apes would be of great importance, if validated. Because neuritic degeneration during aging is found in other nonanthropoid monkeys and pro-simians, its absence in great apes would imply that a canonical neuritic degen-eration of aging re-emerged during recent evolution, possibly in connection with the diet shift. Clearly, a larger number of older great ape brains need to be examined with the currently expanded immunohistochemical battery before firm conclusions can be drawn about the degree of Alzheimer-like neurodegen-

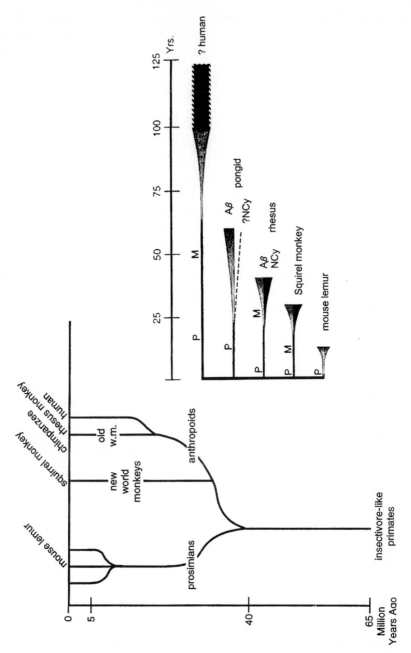

Fig. 1. Primate species Alzheimer-like neurodegeneration. Further developed from Finch and Sapolsky (1999). Thickening of the horizontal lines approximate the incidence of amyloid β-peptide deposits (Aβ) and neurocytoskeletal abnormalities (NCy), which indicate Alzheimer-like neurodegeneration. P, puberty; M, menopause in females where observed (no menopause evident in mouse lemur and chimpanzee). Pongids (chimpanzees and orangutans) have diffuse deposits of Aβ but have not shown NCy (chimpanzee, 56 and 59 years); orangutan (21–46 years).

eration in the great apes. While these modest amyloid accumulations (plaques and vascular amyloid) would not suffice for a histopathologic diagnosis of AD by human criteria, they nonetheless clearly share the amyloid component of the Alzheimer processes that occurs widely in aging humans, nonhuman primates (Fig. 1), and certain other mammals (Finch and Sapolsky 1999).

Nothing is known about neuron cell numbers during aging in the great apes. No neuron loss was found in aging rhesus monkeys aged 24 years, when other studies showed extensive neuritic plaques and memory impairments (Merrill et al. 2001); this study emphasized the entorhinal cortex region; which is a major target of AD (Gomez-Isla et al. 1996).

In general, neuron loss in adult brains is increasingly regarded as a change due to AD or other specific disease processes that are distinct from normal aging (Merrill et al. 2001; West et al. 1994). However, as indicated by the observations in aging rhesus, cognitive impairments during aging may arise independently of neuron loss. Further direct support of this finding comes from studies on aging rats, in which subgroups with impaired memory showed no difference in neuron numbers (Rasmussen et al. 1996). Moreover, in transgenic mice that carry human AD genes, impaired memory correlated best with the amount of soluble $A\beta$ (Mucke et al. 2000). Soluble $A\beta$ includes oligomers of $A\beta 1-42$, which are designated amyloid-derived diffusible ligands (ADDLs; Lambert et al. 1998). ADDLs impair LTP, a neurophysiological function related to memory, and can be neurotoxic, as observed by an author of this paper (CEF) in collaboration with William Klein and Grant Krafft (Oda et al. 1995; Klein et al. 2001; Lambert et al. 1998, 2001). ADDLs are also found in human AD brains (Lambert et al. 2001). It may be possible to obtain frozen specimens from brains of aging pongids within the 6- to 12-hour postmortem interval that allows detection of ADDLs in human AD brains. The presence of ADDLs could be more indicative of cognitive impairments during aging than the amount of neuritic or neurofibrillary degeneration in nonhuman primates.

Future research promises to distinguish various processes of brain aging that can be detected in midlife in clinically normal individuals, e.g., the strong progressive trend toward impaired eye-blink conditioning that shows a linear decline across adult life, long before there is any accumulation of amyloid or neuritic degeneration (Woodruff-Pak and Thompson 1988). Similar changes occur during middle age in rabbits, which do not normally develop amyloid deposits during aging (Woodruff-Pak et al. 1987, 1988). However, some cognitive and behavioral characteristics of young adults are associated with increased risk of AD; we have several important examples, with effect ranges of about 2.5-fold: writers of essays with limited informational and emotional content had a higher risk of AD in later years (Nun Study; Danner et al. 2001; Snowdon et al. 1996) and those with decreased intellectual activities had a higher risk from early to middle adulthood (Friedland et al. 2001).

Selection for Slower Aging and Multigenerational Support

Middle-age features of brain aging would be sensitive to natural selection in long-lived human ancestors who, if they were like hunter-gatherers, achieved peak productivity in their thirties. In the brilliant analysis of Kaplan et al. (2000), the hunter-gatherers do not reach their peak productivity until late in their fourth decade, whereas peak productivity in chimpanzees is acquired soon after weaning. As argued by Finch and Sapolsky (1999), an emerging suite of characteristics would select for genes that delay the age of onset of myocardial and cognitive dysfunctions. In particular, the prolongation of postnatal dependency is proposed to be associated with learning of increasingly efficacious strategies for hunting and gathering and the manufacture and use of tools. Impairments of myocardial or cognitive functions would be selected against in this new cultural regime. Moreover, this selection regime may have been operating for a long time, in view of the trends in anthropoid evolution for fewer offspring and increasingly prolonged postnatal care. For example, Alzheimer-type pathology in the prosimian mouse lemur arises by six years; if this schedule persisted, chimpanzees would already be impaired by the age of sexual maturity (Fig. 1).

Multigenerational interactions are also widely posited to be of increasing importance for transfer of information from the experience of elders. We would add assistance during birth to this suite of social support. Unassisted birth is the norm in the great apes, which generally have no difficulty in labor and parturition (Abitbol 1996). In contrast, the much larger head of the term human infant causes great difficulties during labor, which is often prolonged. Unassisted birthing is very dangerous to mother and child. An analysis of pelvic anatomy of Lucy (*Australopithecus afarensis*, 3 mya) in relation to the head size of *Pan* (chimpanzee) or other hominids suggests major difficulties in birth: "...*serious dystocia problems in view of her narrow antero-posterior diameters at the level of each pelvic plane... If a modern human with a [similar] pelvis carried a fetus of similar dimension [to] Pan, she would require a cesaerian section, deliver a markedly traumatized infant, or die in childbirth.*" (Abitbol 1996, pp 147–148). Thus, the sharp increase in head size would be another factor in multigenerational care giving that emerged at about the same time as increased meat eating.

Meat Eating

Chimpanzees

Meat eating is not the norm for the anthropoid primates. The diet of most higher primates consists largely of leaves and fruit, and foraging for these consumes most of their waking hours. Although the components of these herbivorous dietary generalists vary greatly between taxa, it is widely thought that the diet of anthropoid ancestors in the Miocene was a generalized frugivory (Andrews 1981). As shown by the dental structures of Miocene fossils (> 20 mya), many earlier anthropoids evolved specializations, such as the lengthening of shearing crests for folivery or in the thickness of dental enamel for feeding on hard objects such as nuts (Ungar and Kay 1995).

The main exception to herbivory is the eating of mammalian meat by humans and chimpanzees. The gorilla and bonobo exclusively feed on fruit, leaves, and nuts. As our closest living relative (Ruvolo et al. 1991; Horai et al. 1992), the chimpanzee gives a key precedent for the use of meat by early hominids, which suggests an evolutionary path for the origins of meat-eating in the human lineage. We note that variable amounts of termite larvae and other insects are also commonly eaten by chimpanzees, as well as by orangutans and gorillas. It is possible that the dental specializations of extant or fossil apes facilitate eating of insects.

Recent data show routine hunting by chimpanzees in a variety of environments (Goodall 1986; Boesch and Boesch 1989; Stanford et al. 1994; Stanford 1998). While mainly frugivorous, the quantity of mammalian meat eaten by wild chimpanzees can exceed 0.5 kg/week/individual, as an annual average (Stanford 1998). Nonetheless, the chimpanzee level of meat consumption is much lower than that documented in human foragers (Cordain et al. 2001, 2002 a). In particular, there is no evidence that animal meat is essential for normal pregnancy or nursing (Goodall 1986; Stanford 1998). As observed in some, but not all, chimpanzee communities, meat from captured *Colubus* monkeys and other small prey is used in a social context by males, including attracting females (Stanford 1998, 1999). Overall, males capture about four-fold more prey than females; there are no quantitative data on sex differences in total meat consumed.

The organ preference of chimpanzees includes the brain, which is a potential source of harmful viruses (Sharp et al. 2001; Liberski and Gajdusek 1997). We consider this organ preference important because the brain is a source of fat in all seasons, while fats are typically scarce in plant materials (Cordain et al. 2002 a). Another source of fat in chimpanzees and probably other great apes is insect larvae, which vary seasonally. Examination of fecal content indicates that females consume two-fold more insects and other invertebrates than males (McGrew 1992).

Meat and Fat in Human Diets

Reconstructions of early hominid behavior have been based on diet since Dart (1953). The evolutionary history of meat eating is hard to trace, because most of the meat eaten by chimpanzees is in the form of small mammals, whose remains leave few archeological traces (Stanford 1998). Most archeologists recognize that social behavior and organization depend on the need to balance energy output with nutrient energy intake. The highly concentrated nutrients and calories in meat may have provided emerging humans with nutritional supplements that favored the evolution of other key traits. Meat-eating is thus considered to be the most critical dietary adaptation in human evolution (Stanford and Bunn 2001). Early humans were eager omnivores, at least by 2.5 mya, as indicated by evidence of the manufacture and use of stone tools and associations with human-made cutmarks on fossil remains (Shipman 1986; Bunn and Kroll 1986; Asfaw et al. 1999). Meat was likely obtained through both hunting (Stiner 2001; Speth and Tchernov 2001) and scavenging (Blumenschine 1987).

The consumption of large amounts of protein from any source appears to require sufficient intake of fat and carbohydrate to enable production of urea by the liver (Rudman et al. 1973). As amino acids are catabolized, ammonia is produced by deamidation. Under normal conditions, the liver detoxifies the ammonia through the urea cycle. But the production of urea is coupled to the input of aspartate through the citric acid cycle, which in turn is fed by catabolites of fat and carbohydrates. Diets that are rich in lean-meat and diets with low or negligible carbohydrate and fat can cause a toxic syndrome of protein poisoning associated with ultimately fatal blood levels of ammonia and amino acids (Speth 1989, 1991; Cordain et al. 2002 b).

With the ingestion of increasing amounts of protein at fixed amounts of carbohydrate and fat, 190 g of protein was estimated to provide maximal urea synthesis (Rudman et al. 1973). In two recent studies of healthy young men, a 250 % increase in protein intake produced similar increases in urea production (Forslund et al. 1998) during fasting, feeding, and nocturnal phases (Forslund et al. 1999). Exercise further increased urea production at both protein levels (Forslund et al. 1999). We do not know if the maximal urea production estimated by Rudman et al. (1973) might be increased by further supplements of carbohydrate or fat. These findings provide ample basis for the prediction for ancient humans that, in seasons when prey animals were lean and vegetation sources were low, energetic demands for meat protein would also have motivated the consumption of fat from brain and bone marrow, just as is observed in huntergatherers (Speth 1983, 1989).

The kidney can also limit protein consumption. On one hand, many studies of rodents have shown that high protein diets increase chronic renal disease, particularly the glomerulonephritis that is common in aging laboratory rodent colonies (Finch 1990). On the other hand, a common clinical treatment for human renal insufficiency is to lower protein intake (Zarazaga et al. 2001). Similarly, caloric restriction greatly slows the progression of glomerulonephritis in lab rodents (Finch 1990). It is plausible that the major increase in protein in paleohuman diets also selected for kidney function.

There are many unknowns about the role of dietary fats in supporting or enabling human brain evolution and normal brain development. A valuable series of papers by Cordain, Eaton and colleagues emphasizes that meat eating greatly increases access to fat, and fat is very low in plant materials (e.g., Eaton et al. 1998; Cordain et al. 2002 a). Clearly, brain lipids increase markedly during the last trimester and first postnatal year, but how diet supports optimum development is not clear. Brain maturation is characterized by extensive myelination around cortical neuronal projection pathways, which develops by the successive wrapping around of axons by oligodendroglia. The fatty myelin sheaths produced by the oligodendroglia have a much higher percentage of lipids (70–85 %) than most biological membranes (Morell and Quarles 1999). Myelination enhances the speed of electrical conduction and is crucial to complex cognitive processes. In the more recently evolved higher brain centers, myelination is mostly postnatal and does not approach adult levels until after five years. We do not know in general how human dietary variations in types of fat and fatty acids influence myelination (Crawford 1992; Milton 1999; Innes 2000).

An important gab in understanding concerns the relative importance of dietary versus endogenous synthesis of fatty acids, in particular, the long-chain polyunsaturated fatty acids (PUFAs) that are at low concentrations in plant material (Eaton 1992; Cordain et al. 2002 a). Two widely recognized PUFAs are arachidonic acid (AA) and docosahexaenoic acid (DHA). Both AA and DHA have major roles in regulating membrane functions in brain and other organs. Each is synthesized from a different "essential" fatty acid that may be obtained from the diet. In general, mammals lack enzymes to synthesize PUFAs with double bonds at n-3 or n-6, which is why these PUFAs are designated as "essential" (Innes 2000). AA is synthesized from linoleic acid (18 : 2n-6) and DHA from α-linolenic acid (18 : 3n-3) by further chain elongation (elongases) and desaturation (desaturases), and in the case of linolenic acid, β-oxidases. AA and DHA increase during brain maturation in neuron cell membranes (distinct from myelin).

Under some conditions, deficits of DHA may impair brain and heart functions, although this hypothesis remains highly controversial (British Nutrition Foundation 1992; Innes 2000; Sanders 1999; Ravnskov 1998). Moreover, high levels of brain DHA from diet are associated with auditory and retinal dysfunctions in animal models (Innes 2000).

Both AA and DHA can be synthesized from essential fatty acid precursors by the liver, which releases them into the circulation for uptake by many cell types. Moreover, AA and DHA can be made in the brain by certain cell types. Rat cerebrovascular endothelia and astrocytes, but not neurons, have the required elongases and desaturases (Moore 2001; Williard et al. 2001). In the fetal brain, the synthesis of DHA is sensitive to the ratio of linolenic to α-linoleic acid, because in the test tube, α-linoleic acid competitively inhibits the desaturase required for synthesis of DHA (Sanders 1999). Other unknows include: whether these enzyme activities differ between humans and the anthropoids; how these enzyme activities change during development; and the relative importance of local synthesis versus uptake by brain (Innes 2000; Sanders 1999).

Cordain et al. (2001) concluded that "...*humans maintain an inefficient ability to chain elongate and desaturate fatty acids*". Furthermore "...*the limited availability of these two fatty acids from endogenous metabolic synthesis may have represented the evolutionary bottleneck impeding the encephalization process in all herbivorous mammals. Encephalization quotients decrease with increasing body size because there literally may be insufficient long chain fatty acids (AA and DHA) to build more brain tissues... Cats and other obligate carnivores represent a notable departure from... herbivorous animals because they obtain virtually all of their AA and DHA as preformed product... from their prey"* (Cordain et al. 2001).

It is thus of interest to consider studies of vegetarian women, which showed substantial effects of diet on PUFAs in cord blood of term fetuses and in breast milk (Sanders 1999). In cord blood of term fetuses, DHA was 35 % lower in vegetarians than in omnivores (consistent with the conclusions of Cordain et al. 2002 b), whereas AA was within 10 % in all diet groups. However, the breast milk of vegetarians had about several-fold more linoleic acid (AA precursor) and α-linolenic acid (DHA precursor) than omnivores, which is attributable to their diet. The vegetarians in these studies included a group of vegans, who avoid dairy- and egg-derived food products as well as all vertebrate meat; the vegans had the lowest DHA in breast milk.[1] Sanders (1999) concludes that vegetarians synthesize adequate amounts of AA from linoleic acid; supplements of long chain PUFAs are not absolutely required, unless intake of linoleic acid is excessive, because linoleic acid can inhibit the production of DHA, as noted above.

It is unresolved if human infants should be given dietary supplements of AA and DHA, particularly those given cow's milk which is deficient, relative to human milk, in the essential PUFAs, AA, and DHA (Innes 2000). Postmortem analysis indicates that breast-fed infants had higher DHA than those fed "formula", which may indicate suboptimum intake of DHA (Innes 2000). However, the benefit of supplementing formula with DHA differed between studies of visual functions and of the visual-evoked EEG potential (Sanders 1999).

It is a fair summary of these complex data to say that there is no consensus on the optimum dietary intake of PUFA and other fats for human development and for adult health. It is timely to consider gene expression profiling in different brain cell types of chimpanzees versus humans for various sets of genes that mediate fat metabolism (discussed below).

Cholesterol Sensitivity and Vascular Disease in Chimpanzees

Chimpanzees are remarkably sensitive to diet-induced hypercholesterolemia. In the development of primate models for vascular disease, the great apes have been less widely studied because of cost. Most studies have used smaller species such as baboons, macaques and squirrel monkeys, which also chimpanzees

---

[1] The vegan diet is not comparable to that of the great apes because of its typically high content of cultivated grains. Maize and corn oil, for example, are rich in linoleic acid (AA precursor), which can induce immune dysfunctions if diet is uncompensated for other PUFA (Sammon 1999).

Table 3. Serum chemistry, normative values[a]

	Chimpanzee, control diets	Gorilla, control diets	Human
Copper and iron	= human (Planas and Grau 1971)	= human (Planas and Grau 1971)	
Cholesterol: phospholipid	= human (Peeters and Blaton 1972)		
Total cholesterol (mg/dl)	160–280	272 ± 85 (5) (Nelson et al. 1984)	160–200, normal; 350, type II hyperlipoproteinemia
	259 ± 21 (4) (Blaton et al. 1974); 185 ± 12 (4, M) (Rosseneu et al. 1979)[b]		
	168 ± 30 (15, F) 157 ± 25 (13, M) (Doucet et al. 1994)[c]		
	203 ± 48 (43) (Nelson et al. 1984)		
	248 ± 64 (5, F-lean) 232 ± 55 (13, F-fat) (Steinetz et al. 1996)		

[a] Mean ± SEM (# animals; sex, if given)
[b] Both reports are from the same research group in Belgium
[c] Doucet et al. (1994) report slightly lower values for total cholesterol and HDL cholesterol than in humans, which may be due to diet (see text).

respond. Chimpanzees are of particular value for such studies because their lipoprotein classes are considered identical to those of humans (Steinetz et al. 1996). In general the blood chemistry of chimpanzees and gorillas is very close to that of humans (Table 3). A general view is that blood cholesterol in these species shows greater response to diet than humans. At the other extreme, domestic cats and dogs are considered resistant to diet-induced hypercholesterolemia and vascular disease (see Wissler and Vesselinovitch 1968). These species differences may be of great importance, because canids and felines are carnivores, with evidence in their clades of long-standing meat adaptation, whereas the anthropoids have been largely vegetarian, as noted above.

We briefly note that all studies of captive pongids must be weighed in terms of intrinsic confounds. The amount of exercise is clearly important and rarely addressed. Even in colonies that allow semi-freedom, chimpanzees still have much less daily exercise than feral chimpanzees, which routinely traverse > 5 kms of forest per day while foraging (Wrangham 1975; Goodall 1986). The linear distances traversed do not indicate the effort required, as known by anyone who has tracked animals through uneven bushy terrain. We speak from personal experience. As another perspective, hunter-gatherers are estimated to burn > 5-fold more kcal/kg/day than sedentary office workers (Cordain et al. 1997, 1998). The lack of exercise can adversely affect vascular functions and blood lipids in humans, as well as in captive and wild populations of other primates (see Clarkson et al. 1987; Sapolsky and Mott 1987).

Another factor is the artificial diet provided, which often includes variable amounts of atypical nutrients such as fish and milk products and animal fat that are not ingested in the wild (see details in two studies discussed below). These abnormal (xenotropic) constituents could cause food allergies that might not be obvious. The wide range of individual cholesterol values in captive chimpanzees (Vastesaeger et al. 1972; Steinetz 1996) could also reflect unknown degrees of stress from social isolation or social hierarchy. Nonetheless, the limited literature on captive pongids is consistent in concluding that pongids are highly sensitive to diet-induced hyperlipidemia and vascular lesions.

On various low fat "nonatherogenic diets", captive chimpanzees and gorillas tend to have higher basal serum total cholesterol than normative human values, but studies vary widely, as surveyed in Table 3. Two recent detailed studies give remarkably different profiles of blood lipids that may be due to particular diet and housing conditions. On one hand, uniformly low blood cholesterol was observed in a chimpanzee colony in Gabon Africa (Region Centre for Training and Research in Human Reproduction). Animals were "... *maintained on a classic vegetarian diet with fruits and vegetable supplemented with Cerelac (750 ml/day)... in semi-freedom...*" (Doucet et al. 1994).[2] In this colony, total and LDL cholesterol were "... *slightly but significantly lower...*" in chimpanzees (N = 28, aged 6–19 years) than in healthy adult humans (N = 27). However, chimpanzees showed slightly elevated triglycerides. Two animals with outlying values were excluded (one with high triglycerides, the other with low apoB-100).

In contrast to this study, another population showed a much greater proportion of high blood lipid values – the large (former) colony at LEMSIP (N.Y.U.; Steinetz et al. 1996). Adult chimpanzees aged about 25 years were fed ad libitum a "low fat" diet.[3] It is of great interest to note that hypercholesterolemia was rampant in this colony, relative to the Gabonese chimpanzees, and occurred in both lean and obese individuals (Table 3; 50 % of obese and 30 % of

---

[2] Cerelec (Nestlé Inc.) is a maize-milk weaning food.

[3] The named diet, Jumbo Monkey Diet 5037 (Steinetz et al. 1996), appears to be the Purina (PMI Feeds Inc.) Monkey Diet No. 5037, packaged as "Jumbo" biscuits and designed for Old Worlds monkeys. Its components include cultivated grains and soybean, whey (milk component presumably from cows), fish meal, and animal fat. Although the proportions of bulk proteins, fats, and carbohydrates may vary within narrow limits (as specified for this Purina product), the specific sources of most commercial diets can vary seasonally by bulk availability and market price, particularly for fish meal and animal fat; these variations may be important because of trace components that can be allergenic. Purina guarantees for diet no. 5037 that crude protein is at least 15 % and crude fat at least 5 % (PMI description, 2001). The composition listed by Steinetz et al. (1996, Table 1) shows 15.5 % protein and 10.9 % fat. The latter value indicates that fat content can vary at least two-fold in food lots, which could cause differences in blood lipid values.

lean individuals), which reached the criteria for type II hyperlipidemia (LDL-cholesterol > 160 mg/dl, the National Cholesterol Education Program guidelines). We quote these authors: *"The chimpanzee thus appears to be superior to many other animal models [for vascular disease]... abnormal lipid values were achieved without recourse to an atherogenic diet"* (Steinetz et al. 1996). It is also cogent that adult chimpanzees in this population had a high incidence of obesity (> 90 % of females sampled); these authors suggested that the sedentary lifestyle of captive chimpanzees might be a factor in the lipid abnormalities of the obese individuals. In natural populations, obesity is rarely observed, although females become heavier in the rainy season (Wrangham 1975).

We may conclude that in optimal conditions, which may be approximated by the Doucet et al. (1994) study, captive chimpanzees have in low incidence of hyperlipidemia, but that hyperlipidemia is readily induced on diets and under husbandry conditions that are considered nonatherogenic for other primates (Steinetz et al. 1996). Note that neither study used a completely typical diet eaten by feral adult chimpanzees, which would never include the grains or milk components of the Cerelac and Purina diets (see footnotes 2 and 3). It would be of great value to know the blood lipid profiles of feral chimpanzees, especially in relation to the consumption of meat, which varies widely between individuals and communities. It may be possible to obtain some information on cholesterol from feces (Mann 1972). (In certain African countries, excreta are the only materials allowed for biological sampling in feral endangered species.)

Consistent with the conclusions of Steinetz et al. (1996), several studies of atherogenic diets conclude that chimpanzees are more sensitive to diet-induced hypercholesterolemia than most other nonhuman primates, as well as humans. According to two, long-term dietary studies, chimpanzees are about four-fold more sensitive to increased dietary cholesterol than humans or baboons. The most detailed reports are from a decade-long study at the Simon Steven Institute in Brugge, Belgium (Blaton et al. 1970, 1972, 1974 a, b; Howard et al. 1972; Peeters et al. 1970; Rosseneu et al. 1979; Vastesaeger et al. 1972; see calculations in footnote 3)[4]. Similarly, Mann and colleagues at Vanderbilt University also concluded that chimpanzees have a four-fold greater sensitivity to increased dietary cholesterol than humans; this single report, which appears to summarize extensive studies, also gives values for other mammals (Mann 1964).

Consistent with the blood lipid profile, chimpanzees are considered to be relatively more vulnerable to spontaneous and diet-induced aortic and cerebral atherosclerosis than other nonhuman primates (Andrus et al. 1968; Blaton et al. 1972 a, b; Ratcliffe 1965). One young adult female had an initial blood cholesterol level of 400 mg/dl, which is within the upper range of captive chimpanzees on control diets, and, after receiving the atherogenic diet for a few months died

---

[4] In Blaton et al. (1972 a, the same atherogenic diet increased total plasma cholesterol in the chimpanzee four times more than in the baboon; basal [B] vs atherogenic [A] diet, values in mg cholesterol/dl serum: chimpanzee, B, 259 vs A, 606, net increase of 347; baboon, B 117 vs A, 203, net increase of 86; whence, 347 [chimp.]) 86 (baboon) = 4.03-fold greater increment in chimpanzee than baboon.

"unexpectedly" from a large coronary infarction (Vastesaeger et al. 1972). During two years on a high cholesterol diet, another young female had total cholesterol up to 900 mg/dl (upper clinical range for hyperlipidemia) and also died *"unexpectedly"*; autopsy and histopathology showed a recent myocardial infarction and distributed atheromatous lesions extending to the cerebral arteries (briefly described in Blaton et al. 1972; full description in Vastesaeger et al. 1972). Mann (1972) concluded that *"Chimpanzees [are] exceptionally sensitive to dietary cholesterol – ranking with the rabbit . . . and may be the most prone of all primates to atherosclerosis"*.

The cholesterol sensitivity of chimpanzees has not been considered in relation to the intake of mammalian meat observed in many feral anthropoid populations. There is no information on how meat consumption might influence life expectancy. Moreover, we lack information on causes of spontaneous death in adult chimpanzees apart from those caused by fighting or accidental injury. In view of the deaths from myocardial infarction observed in relatively young captive chimpanzees, it is possible that vascular disease in association with meat eating is a factor in morbidity and mortality.

The much lower threshold level for dietary cholesterol on blood hypercholesterolemia in chimpanzees than humans could limit the reproductive potential of male chimpanzees by increasing their risk of mortality from heart attacks or strokes. It seems plausible that humans have evolved genes that allow much greater intake of meat than in stem-line anthropoid ancestors. Mann and colleagues (same as Mann 1972 above) examined the Masai of east Africa, who are pastoralists; their traditional diet is mostly meat, milk, and blood, with less regular intake of vegetables (Mann and Shaffer 1966; Dock 1971). Despite this atherogenic diet, Masai men have a low incidence of hyperlipidemia, coronary disease, and hypertension (Mann 1964, Mann et al. 1972; Ho et al. 1971). Even in pregnancy, when blood cholesterol typically increases up to two-fold by the 30th week, the women did not have elevated blood cholesterol, which remained about 150 mg/dl throughout (Mann and Shaffer 1966). The very high level of aerobic conditioning in Masai men may be a factor in their resistance to heart disease on diets associated in other populations with hypercholesterolemia (Mann et al. 1965). It would in interesting to follow-up these observations of four decades ago with comparisons of urbanized and traditional Masai.

Lastly, we note the broad commonality of humans with other anthropoids in showing early stage vascular lesions as vigorous young adults. Preatherosclerotic lesions were common, for example, in US soldiers killed in Korea and Vietnam (Mann et al. 1971; Leistikow 1998; also, Finch and Kirkwood 2000, p. 195). Further development into occlusive vascular conditions, however, appears to depend on ecological or lifestyle variable that include diet, exercise, and stress, as indicated for both humans and the great apes as discussed above. The basic pathophysiological mechanisms of vascular disease seem shared across the anthropoids, with important species differences in the degree of sensitivity to dietary fat.

Cholesterol and Alzheimer's Disease (AD)

Human Studies of AD Incidence

Elevated cholesterol is also emerging as a risk factor in AD in population surveys and from animal models (Simons et al. 2001; Wolozin 2001; Wolozin et al. 2000; Marx 2001). To summarize an emerging and, of course, somewhat inconsistent literature, subgroups of several populations with high consumption of animal fat and/or low consumption of fish have a 50–100 % higher incidence of AD (Mayeux et al. 1999; Deschamps et al. 2001; Kalmijn 2000; Newman 1998).

Other evidence concerns statins, which have come into widespread use to lower blood cholesterol. In several large studies of statins, users who were being treated prospectively for vascular risk factors had a 70 % lower risk of AD (Jick et al. 2000; Wolozin et al. 2000). Statins inhibit cholesterol synthesis HMG-CoA reductase and can cross the blood-brain barrier to act on brain cells. However, statins also act on inflammatory mechanisms that are also involved in AD. Conversely, elevated cholesterol at midlife increases the risk of AD and other cognitive impairments (Notkola et al. 1998; Kivipelto et al. 2001).

In a study by Wolozin et al. (2000), AD prevalence in patients 60 years or older was evaluated in databases from three US hospitals (Chicago region: Loyola University Medical Center, 22,143 records, and Edward Hines Jr VA Hospital, 23,028 records; Phoenix region, Carl T Hayden VA Medical Center Ariz, 15,178 records). One group received several statins [lovastatin (Mevacor), pravastatin (Pravachol), and simvastatin (Zocor)]; another group received other (nonstatin) drugs for hypertension or cardiovascular disease. Those who received lovastatin or pravastatin showed a 73 % lower AD prevalence than those taking beta-blockers: 64 % less than captopril, and 57 % less than furosemide. These comparisons are valuable controls for possible referral biases. (Some clinicians hesitate to request neurological examinations of possible dementia in those with hypertension who are at risk for stroke, which also causes dementia.) Jick et al. (2000) used a case-control method to examine a General Practice Research Database in England. Patients aged 50 and older who received statins were compared with hyperlipidemic patients not treated with statins (N = 284) and with random control (N = 1080). Statin users showed a 71 % lower risk of AD, in remarkable agreement with Wolozin et al. (2000).

Cholesterol and Amyloid in Animal Models

Animal models show even more convincing effects of cholesterol. Feeding of cholesterol increases brain amyloid deposits, first shown in rabbits (Sparks 1996) and recently extended to transgenic mice that carry human familial AD genes (Refolo et al. 2001). Moreover, guinea pigs treated with statins have lower Aβ peptide in their cerebrospinal fluid (Fassbender et al. 2001). The mechanism appears to involve the cholesterol levels in brain membranes where the amyloid precursor protein (APP) is processed to the Aβ peptide (Simons et al. 2001; Mills and Reiner 1999). Membrane cholesterol increases can enhance production of Aβ peptide by inhibiting the predominant "non-amyloidgenic" α-secretase pathway of APP processing and enhancing the minor β-secretase "amyloidogenic" pathway (Riddell et al. 2001; Kojro et al. 2001).

Cholesterol esters are another candidate in AD prevention, particularly those in the cytoplasmic pool regulated by acyl-coenzymeA: cholesterol acyl transferase (ACAT). Decreases of membrane cholesterol are replaced by hydrolysis of cholesterol esters; conversely, increased free cholesterol activates ACAT and increases the cytoplasmic depots of cholesterol esters. Puglielli et al. (2001) showed that ACAT activity modulates APP processing in neurons and other cells with positive correlations between the levels of cholesterol esters and Aβ production. The APP secretases are modulated by cholesterol ester levels and cultured neurons were particularly sensitive. Several ACAT inhibitors used to treat atherosclerosis, e.g., CL277, 082, and melinamide, might also benefit AD risk.

A converse of cholesterol feeding or statin treatment may be found in caloric restriction, which increases rodent life span (Sohal and Weindruch 1996; Finch 1990; Patel and Finch 2002). In Alzheimer-transgenic mice, caloric restriction of adult mice by a standard protocol (35% restriction of ad lib) appeared to slow the accumulation of amyloid deposits (Connor et al. 2000; Patel, Morgan, Finch, unpublished). Although there is no information on whether caloric restriction modifies brain cholesterol, caloric restriction slightly lowers total blood cholesterol in rats (Van Liew et al. 1993). This finding may not be relevant to brain, which synthesizes much of its own cholesterol.

Cholesterol and Tau Phosphorylation

Cholesterol may also influence the neurofibrillary tangles (NFT), the intraneuronal aggregates of hyperphosphorylated tau that are a characteristic of AD, besides the extracellular amyloid plaques. Neuronal cholesterol in AD brains was recently quantified by filipin histochemistry and shows a small increase of 1–2% in NFT-bearing neuron vs adjacent normal neurons (Distl et al. 2001). There is reason to consider that these subtle changes in cholesterol are cause rather than effect, because of the NFT in Niemann-Pick type C (NPC) disease, which is an autosomal recessive disease with characteristic cholesterol accumulations in many organs. Lowdensity, lipoprotein-derived cholesterol accumulates because of defective cholesterol trafficking from lysosomes. The brain shows progressive neurodegeneration, with neurofibrillary tangles (NFT) and neuron death. Remarkably, no amyloid deposits are found. Moreover, neurons of NPC brains showed activation of mitogen-activated protein kinase, which can phosphorylate tau (Sawamura et al. 2001). The higher systemic cholesterol levels of apoE4 carriers thus could independently contribute to tau hyperphosphorylation and to amyloid plaques. The absence of plaques in NPC indicates that several pathways are at work in AD.

Two other types of observations appear to give opposite effects of choles-terol. In cultured neurons (Fan et al. 2001) or brain slices (Bi et al. 2001; Koudi-nova and Koudinova 2001), decreased intracellular cholesterol caused a range of neuronal dysfunction that overlap with AD, including increased tau phosphory-lation, destabilized microtubules, and axonal degeneration. These responses to lower cholesterol appear to be proAD and opposite to the effects of lower cellu-lar cholesterol in inhibiting production of Aβ described above. Moreover, total starvation of mice for one to three days caused progressive increases in hippo-campal tau phosphorylation; refeeding reversed these effects within one day (Yanagisawa et al. 1999). There is no information on how starvation to near the point of death in mice may alter particular pools of cholesterol in the brain. It seems likely that different subcellular cholesterol pools could independently regulate microtubule phosphorylation and the APP secretases.

Candidate Genes

The Meat-Adaptive Genes of Lipoprotein Metabolism

The major increase in meat eating during human evolution would also promote vascular disease and AD though the increased blood levels of cholesterol and triglycerides. As previously noted, the consumption of high levels of protein requires a sufficient intake of fat and carbohydrate to drive the urea cycle and avoid protein poisoning from excess production of ammonia and free amino acids. Thus, high-energy meat diets would be coupled to increased levels of blood cholesterol. Sex differences may be important in relation to the greater meat consumption of males to support arduous hunting expeditions (this may be anticipated by the greater activity in male chimpanzees in hunting).

If early *Homo* had the same sensitivity to hyperlipidemias and vascular dis-ease as described above for chimpanzees, few adults would have been healthy in their thirties, when hunter-gatherers are achieving peak productivity (Kaplan et al. 2000). These changes in diet occurred over a span of several million years, during which time we propose there was natural selection for resistance to hyperlipidemias in young and middle-aged adults. The increased intake of mammalian brain and liver would also have increased levels of intake of arachi-donic acid (AA) and docosahexaenoic acid (DHA), which are postulated to pro-mote encephalization. The evolution of resistance to adverse effects of meat pre-dicts a functional class of genes that we designate as "meat-adaptive genes".

Clues about the identity of meat-adaptive genes can be drawn from the genetics of lipoprotein abnormalities associated with heart disease. In his useful review of this huge field, Breslow (2000) summarizes evidence that three blood components are independent risk factors in vascular disease: elevations of LDL cholesterol and triglycerides increase risk, whereas elevations of HDL choles-terol reduce risk. More than 50 genes regulate blood cholesterol and triglycer-ides. The most extreme dysfunctions are associated with rare familial mutations, e.g., in the familial hyperlipidemias traced to mutant LDL receptors. Some of genes have variants that are more common, e.g., heterozygosity for a particular LDL receptor defect is present in 0.02 % of the population in association with two-fold elevations of plasma LDL cholesterol. But at the population level, familial genes with extreme phenotypes may account for < 10 % of adult-onset vascular pathology. *A working hypothesis is that most variations in blood lipids derive from combinations of milder genetic variants, with many environmental influences (diet, exercise, stress), which give "context-dependent" genetic effects.*

Apolipoprotein E, Alzheimer's Disease, and Cholesterol

Humans

The main genetic risk factor of coronary artery disease appears to be the fairly common ε4 allele of apolipoprotein E *(apoE4)*, which subsequently has been shown to be a common risk factor for AD, as discussed below. The apoE allele system is associated with about 10 % of the variance in blood cholesterol, with *E4/E4* genotypes having the highest blood cholesterol. Overall, *E4/E4* accelerates AD risk by 15 years and appears to intensify oxidative stress and other aspects of neurodegeneration. We will argue that apoE was a target of selection for increased vascular and cognitive health at middle age, because only humans have the ApoE3 isoform. ApoE alleles are being implicated in many other effects of broad importance to neurological diseases and beyond, e.g., apoE4 was associated with reduced male fecundity and increased risk of birth defects (Gerdes et al. 1996). These and other examples are discussed in Finch and Sapolsky (1999) and Bedlack et al. (2000).

The ancestral allele is the health-endangering apoE4 allele, the only isoform found in all primates examined (Finch and Sapolsky 1999; Mahley and Rall 2000), as first indicated from restriction fragment length polymorphisms (RFLP; Hanlon and Rubensztein 1995; see summary in Finch and Sapolsky 1999, Table 4). This hypothesis was substantiated by direct sequencing of one chimpanzee apoE gene and comparisons with many human genes (Fullerton et al. 2000). Analysis of the gene sequence in four ethnic groups (4951 nt; African-Americans, Mayans, Finns, and non-Hispanic whites, N = 48 per group) showed 31 distinct *apoE* haplotypes (22 variable sites; Fullerton et al. 2000). The human consensus sequence has 76 differences from the chimpanzee (63 nt substitutions; 13 length differences up to 36 nt). The time of divergence (equivalent to expansion of an ancestral allele) is in the range of 200,000–300,000 years (226,000 years with 95 % credibility intervals 175,000–600,000 years), assuming a constant molecular clock. Most of the human intra-allelic divergence appears to be within the past 60,000 years. Fullerton et al. (2000) calculated that the time depth of human apoE does not differ significantly from human β-globin, a neutral autosomal locus with an age of

770,000 and a broad confidence range of 420,000 years. Although the analysis of Fullerton et al. (2000) cannot inform about selective advantages for the newly evolved *apoE3* and *apoE2*, many studies show consistent disadvantages of *apoE4* to health during aging.

Most human populations show an increased risk of AD in *apoE4* carriers with allele dose dependency (Farrer et al. 1997; Roses 1998; Poirier 2000). However, African-Americans and Latin Americans do not consistently show *apoE4* allele dose effects on AD risk (Stewart et al. 2001; Tang et al. 1998; Farrer et al. 1997). A particularly interesting comparison is of community-dwelling African-Americans in Indianapolis and Yoruba in Ibadan Nigeria (Hendrie et al. 2001). This longitudinal, community-based study examined nearly 5,000 elderly individuals with a 5-year later follow-up. Evaluation was based on an interview test designed to detect memory impairments across cultural diversity and educational levels. The incidence of dementia was about 70 % lower in the elderly Yoruba than in the African-Americans. The incidence of apoE4 was identical in both populations and was only weakly associated with dementia in the African-Americans and not at all in the Yoruba. Although the ancestors of African-Americans in Indianapolis is not known, it is possible that some were Yoruba, since this region of Nigeria was a major source of slaves brought to the New World (Thomas 1997). The Yoruba have a lower incidence of vascular disease, diabetes, and hypertension, and lower blood cholesterol (references in Hendrie et al. 2001). The typical diet of the Muslim Yoruba in Ibadan is characterized as low in fat and protein, consisting mostly of yam and casava, with some corn and fish (Hugh C Hendrie, personal communication; Adeoye 1992). The low dietary fat and low incidence of AD are consistent with fat being a risk factor for AD in other human and animal model studies reviewed above. The variations between populations may reflect statistical interactions of blood cholesterol levels with apoE alleles. Another study of African-Americans showed a greater risk of AD in *apoE4* carriers who had low cholesterol; in *apo2* or *apoE3* carriers, total cholesterol showed a linear effect on AD risk, which converged to the same risk at higher cholesterol levels (Evans et al. 2000).

ApoE4 is showing associations with cognitive deficits, in the absence of clinical AD. Nondemented *apoE4* carriers at middle age show lower glucose utilization in brain regions affected during AD (Small et al. 2000; Reiman et al. 1996). Lower metabolism predicted cognitive decline during the next two years; although the *apoE4* carriers did not differ at the beginning of the study in cognitive test performance, they did have complaints about mild memory impairments for recalling names and misplacing familiar objects. Mild cognitive impairments might be disadvantageous to the rigorous demands of hunter-gatherers. Because this sample was mostly Caucasian (Small et al. 2000), data on African-Americans would be of much greater interest in view of their weaker association of AD with *apoE4*.

ApoE isoforms also influence cholesterol responses so diet and exercise (reviewed by Tikkanen et al. 1995; Hagberg et al. 2000). *ApoE4* increases the effects of low-fat diets in reducing plasma LDL and, possibly, the total cholesterol. This greater sensitivity of *apoE4* is consistent with the sensitivity of chimpanzees to hyperlipidemia and vascular disease, because of their *apoE4* genotype. Of particular interest, *apoE4* carriers showed less response to exercise on lowering blood lipids (Tikkanen et al. 1995; Hagberg et al. 2000). We hypothesize that the spread of *apoE3* in human evolution may have been favored by less sensitivity to high-fat diets and increased benefit to those who were highly active, as required by hunter-gatherer lifestyles.

The importance of this interaction could have begun during the prolonged arid phase of 2.5–1.5 mya in East Africa, when there was a shift from woodland to savanna. Cordain et al. (1998) hypothesized that early humans extended their daily range of foraging, and hence their food consumption, during this time. These remarks extend the Finch-Sapolsky (1999) hypothesis that, during human evolution, the emergence of multi-generational social support, including the role of grandmothering, could have extended the duration of active selection against delayed adverse effects to later ages.

Animal Models

ApoE alleles also have important influences on neuropathology in animal models in which the mouse *apoE* gene was knocked-out and replaced by human *apoE3* or *apoE4*. The *apoE4* knock-ins in mice carrying human AD genes (mutant human APP) had greater accumulations of amyloid deposits and poorer performance on memory tests than *apoE3* knock-ins (Carter et al. 2001; Holtzman et al. 2000). Moreover, in a normal background strain mouse not carrying AD genes, the *apoE3* knock-ins performed much better than *apoE4* knock-ins on memory tests (Hartman et al. 2001). This study did not find structural brain abnormalities in a preliminary survey that included levels of the presynaptic protein synaptophysin, which correlates strongly with cognitive impairments in AD. Several labs are looking for abnormalities in brain development in the apoE4 knock-ins, in view of the consistent findings of impaired synaptogenesis in responses to brain lesions in adult humans and animal models (summarized in Finch and Sapolsky 1999 and in many subsequent studies).

Just how *apoE4* enhances the risk of AD is unclear. Multiple mechanisms are likely to be at work because of the multiple functions that this molecule carries out (Mahley and Rall 2000; Finch and Sapolsky 1999). A powerful argument is emerging for the role of brain cholesterol, because increased brain cell cholesterol and cholesterol esters promote formation of the Aβ peptide and possibly its aggregation. As first shown in rabbits, feeding of cholesterol induces accumulations of the Aβ peptide in neurons (Sparks et al. 2000). Moreover, cholesterol feeding accelerates formation of the Aβ deposits in transgenic APP mice (Refolo et al. 2000). Consistent with these in vivo findings, cultured cells produce less Aβ peptide when depleted of cholesterol (Kojro et al. 2001; Riddell et al. 2001). Many labs are studying how cholesterol influences activities of the enzyme systems that regulate APP processing: the α-secretase pathway which cleaves the APP peptide to prevent the formation of the Aβ peptide seems to be inhibited by cholesterol, whereas the β- and γ-secretases which increase Aβ peptide formation are enhanced by cholesterol. As noted above, cholesterol esters and the enzyme ACAT (acyl-coenzymeA: cholesterol acyl transferase) are implicated in these processes (Puglielli et al. 2001). Furthermore, increased cholesterol content of cell surface membranes decreases binding of the Aβ peptide; the decreased binding by cell surfaces could increase concentration in the extracellular space, enhancing the aggregation to neurotoxic forms (Yip et al. 2001).

ApoE isoforms have many other activities that could influence the progression of AD. In the test tube, the formation of aggregates of Aβ is enhanced by *apoE4* more than *by apoE3* (Moir et al. 1999). Moreover, apoE interacts with neurofibrillary tangles (NFTs), which, in AD brains and in the mouse lemur (reviewed in Finch and Sapolsky 1999), include apoE protein. AD brains include a C-terminal fragment of apoE protein, which showed intriguing differences between isoforms (Huang et al. 2001). When introduced into cultured neurons, truncated apoE4 was more active than apoE3 in inducing hyperphosphorylated tau and filamentous inclusion bodies that resembled NFTs.

ApoE, Inflammation, and Host Defense

Lastly, we survey emerging evidence that apoE4 interacts with host defense systems that may be a factor in its maintenance in the gene pool, despite the myriad adverse effects found on aging processes. Charlesworth (1996) may have been the first to suggest that the apoE4 isoform and disease-associated alleles of other genes are maintained in human populations because of some advantage in early life. The enhancement of AD risk during later aging, when selection pressure is greatly decreased, could be an example of "antagonistic pleiotropy", that is, selection of genes for advantages in early life that have delayed adverse consequences at later ages, when reproduction declines and when selection has weakened. Charlesworth did not discuss specific mechanisms.

Several in vitro studies indicate that the apoE4 isoform enhances inflammatory reactions, which might enhance host defense mechanisms against pathogenic organisms. In very recent work by Carol Colton and colleagues, macrophages from normal human E4 carriers and from apoE4 knock-in mice showed enhanced production of free radicals and other inflammatory markers relative to E3 (Brown et al. 2001). Another study showed that apoE4, but not -E3 or -E2, potentiated the activation of complement by Aβ (McGeer et al. 1997).

Postmortem findings from AD brains are consistent with the enhancement of inflammatory processes by apoE4, particularly in the activated microglia around senile plaques, which are known to produce many inflammatory proteins (Akiyama et al. 2000; Finch and Longo 2000). Microglia are derived from bone marrow monocyte lineage cells and resemble macrophages in many regards. Because microglia can produce reactive free radicals, their activation is a potential source of the oxidative damage in AD, which appears to be greater in degenerating brain regions of apoE4 than E3 carriers (Montine et al. 1997; Ramassamy et al. 1999). Just how far these effects extend is not clear. On the other hand, the human apoE3 protein, but not apoE4, blocked the activation of microglia by sAPPα (Barger and Harmon 1997), whereas no isoform differences were found in effects of apoE in attenuating the activation of astrocytes by Aβ (Hu et al. 1998).

The evidence for increased inflammatory responses of apoE4 macrophage-microglia, albeit mixed, still gives a basis for the hypothesis of antagonistic pleiotropy in host resistance, e.g., that the apoE4 allele might have been maintained in human populations by enhancing resistance to many types of infections through the higher inflammatory responses of macrophages, which have a major, immediate role in host-defense. That is, the delayed disadvantages of apoE4 might be outweighed in balancing selection for a better short-term, host defense response. Furthermore, as discussed by Mahley and Rall (2001), HIV and certain other viruses, like apoE, bind to heparin sulfate proteoglycans (HSPG); so far there is no direct evidence that apoE isoforms differentially influence viral binding or uptake by cells. Martin (1999) suggested another mechanism: apoE4 might be a host resistance factor for lipophilic parasites such as trypanosomes, particularly in tropical and equatorial populations where apoE4 tends to have higher prevalence.

There is some evidence that apoE alleles influence infections by viruses and prions. In HIV, apoE4 is associated with a several-fold higher incidence of dementia and peripheral neuropathy (Corder et al. 1998). There is no information on whether apoE alleles influence the risk of infection by HIV. As a case in point, the present HIV epidemic may have originated by ingestion of simian virus relatives found in African chimpanzees (Sharp et al. 2001; Gagneux et al. 2001) through the bush-meat trade or many other types of contact (Gagneux et al. 2001).

Prion diseases may also be sensitive to apoE alleles, but evidence is not consistent. On one hand, Amouyel et al. (1994) found that *apoE4* increased the risk of Creutzfeldt-Jacob disease (CJD), whereas Pickering-Brown et al. (1995) found an association of the *apoE2* with later onset of CJD. The E4 risk of CJD was not confirmed by several other studies (Chapman et al. 1998; Zerr et al. 1996; Nakagawa et al. 1995; Salvatore et al. 1995). Mutations in the host gene PrP^c are a major factor in determining the latency of prion infections and its transmissibility between species (Prusiner and Hsiao 1994). Prion resistance is discussed further below.

Lipoprotein (A)

Blood lipoprotein (a) [Lp(a)] levels are another mild risk factor in vascular disease. High levels of Lp(a) can increase the risk of heart disease by 1.5- to 2-fold (Breslow 2000; Sharrett et al. 2001). In stroke, the effects of Lp(a) levels and apoE4 are independent (Peng et al. 1999).

Chimpanzee Lp(a) is two to four times higher than in humans (Huby et al. 2001), which could be a factor in the sensitivity of chimpanzees to dietary cholesterol. Among humans, genetic differences account for up to 90 % of the individual variations in blood Lp(a) levels, which range > 1000-fold between individuals (Boerwinkle et al. 1992). The basis for the higher level of Lp(a) in chimpanzees was found in a detailed analysis of human and chimpanzee *Lp(a)* genes (Huby et al. 2001). The rates of transcription of the chimpanzee gene were fivefold greater than the human gene, which is an important finding because it indicates that evolutionary changes occurred in gene activity, not in the physiological clearance (turnover) of the blood protein. A functional analysis using site-directed mutagenesis showed that three particular bases in the near-upstream promoter (−3/−2/+8) accounted for the higher transcription rate of chimpanzee *Lp(a)*. The requirement for changes in all three sites to achieve the human rate of gene expression indicates a progressive multistep evolution of the *Lp(a)* gene.

Besides these examples of apoE and Lp(a), many other genes that mediate lipid metabolism are plausible candidates as meat-adaptive genes. In view of the sensitivity of chimpanzees to diet-induced hypercholesterolemia, many candidates from the human genetics of hyperlipidemias may be considered, including the LDL receptor family, some of which are also candidates for AD. Cholesterol esters and the enzyme ACAT are implicated in the processing of the amyloid precursor protein.

Another category of genes is the synthesis of membrane components, e.g., encoding enzymes that synthesize brain fatty acids, arachidonic acid and docosahexaenoic acid, the elongase and desaturases, as discussed previously.

Other Genes

Metal Metabolism

Muscle is also rich in metals (heme-iron, copper and zinc) that can interact with vascular disease and AD. Increased exposure through meat sources would select for enhanced metal storage and detoxification (not discussed here).

Prion Resistance

The prion gene PrP^c is another interesting candidate for selection because of its influence on resistance to prions that may be ingested in raw brain and bone marrow (see above). The gene sequence of humans differs from that of chimpanzees by two amino acids (6 nt) at residues 167 and 171 (Schätzl et al. 1995). The gorilla is even closer, with a single amino acid difference at 168 (glutamate in human; glutamine in gorilla and chimpanzee). These substitutions have not been associated with mutations in human prion diseases; however, other regions of PrP^c influence species barriers to transmission of prion diseases. Host-resistance genes for prion transmission may been of long-standing importance to paleolithic humans who sought marrow and brains (Table 1). For example, Neanderthal cave sites show clear evidence of tool use on fractured long bones and skulls of deer, but also of humans (Defleur et al. 1999). Brains are also eaten by chimpanzees. The prion diseases were first recognized in New Guinea aborigines who ate raw brains of recently decreased relatives (Prusiner et al. 1984; Prusiner and Hsiao 1994; Liberski and Gajdusek 1997). Prions are remarkable among infectious agents for their lack of genomic DNA or RNA, but also for their survival during ordinary cooking. For example, prion infectivity can survive autoclaving at $> 120\,^{\circ}\mathrm{C}$ (Taylor 1999). Thus primitive cooking procedures would not have been likely to eliminate the hazard of infective prions, particularly from ingestion of brain or bone marrow, which were favored targets of paleolithic hunters. Mutations in the PrP^c genes that delay the age of onset (Prusiner et al. 1994; Telling et al. 1996) may have been targets for selection. Primates are recognized for relatively high vulnerability to prion transmission (Schätzl et al. 1995; Cervenáková et al. 1994). This vulnerability is well documented by prion transmission among New Guinea aborigines, in the iatrogenic transmission of Creutzfeldt-Jacob disease from corneal transplants and pituitary growth hormone, and in the mad cow disease of Western Europe (Prusiner et al. 1999).

Differences in Gene Expression

In all of these cases, we must consider not only genetic changes that modify protein structure, as in apoE alleles, but also changes that modify gene expression, as in Lp(a). Gene expression profiling by microarray may be very useful in identifying genes with different levels of expression in humans versus chimpanzees. A preliminary report indicates major differences in mRNA levels between human and chimpanzee brain (Normile 2001).

We suggest an alternative strategy to brute force sequencing of the chimpanzee genome that might elucidate genes that mediated human evolution, particularly in longevity and brain development. For example, chimpanzee and human peripheral blood cells and fibroblasts could be compared by expression profiling quantitative differences in responses to lipids and other dietary constituents, for divalent metalsor for viruses. This physiological genomics strategy would include functional tests by cross-species gene transfection and gene silencing in primary cell cultures. Functional evaluation is not easily devised for most of the chimpanzee-human differences in point mutations or larger rearrangements (Gagneux and Varki 2001).

Acknowledgments

This research was supported by grants to CE Finch from the NIA, the John Douglas French Foundation for Alzheimer's Disease, and the Alzheimer's Association.

References

Abitbol MM (1996) Birth and human evolution: anatomical and obstetrical mechanics in primates. Westport CT, Bergin and Garvy

Adeoye AO (1992) The assessment of nutritional status of a family unit in Idi'kan, Ibadan. Thesis for BS in Dept Human Nutrition, College of Medicine, University of Ibadan, Nigeria. (kindly provided to CEF by HS Hendrie)

Akiyama H, Barger S, Barnum S, Bradt B, Bauer J, Cole GM, Cooper NR, Eikelenboom P, Emmerling M, Fiebich BL, Finch CE, Frautschy S, Griffin WS, Hampel H, Hull M, Landreth G, Lue L, Mrak R, Mackenzie IR, McGeer PL, O'Banion MK, Pachter J, Pasinetti G, Plata-Salaman C, Rogers J, Rydel R, Shen Y, Streit W, Strohmeyer R, Tooyoma I, Van Muiswinkel FL, Veerhuis R, Walker D, Webster S, Wegrzyniak B, Wenk G, Wyss-Coray T (2000) Inflammation and Alzheimer's disease. Neurobiol Aging 21: 383–421

Amouyel P, Vidal O, Launay JM, Laplanche JL (1994) The apolipoprotein E alleles as major susceptibility factors for Creutzfeldt-Jakob disease. The French Research Group on Epidemiology of Human Spongiform Encephalopathies. Lancet 344: 1315–1318

Andrews P (1981) Species diversity and diet in monkeys and apes during the Miocene. In: Stringer C, Aspects of human evolution. London: Taylor & Francis, Ltd, pp. 25–61

Asfaw B, White T, Lovejoy O, Latimer B, Simpson S, Suwa G (1999) Australopithecus garhi: a new species of early hominid from Ethiopia. Science 284: 629–635

Barger SW, Harmon AD (1997) Microglial activation by Alzheimer amyloid precursor protein and modulation by apolipoprotein E. Nature 388: 878–881

Bate AL, Ma JK, Pitt Ford TR (2000) Detection of bacterial virulence genes associated with infective endocarditis in infected root canals. Int Endo J 33: 194–203

Bedlack RS, Strittmatter WJ, Morgenlander JC (2000) Apolipoprotein E and neuromuscular disease: a critical review of the literature. Arch Neurol 57: 1561–1565

Bi X, Zhou J, Sharman K, Song Z, Liu J, Lynch G (2001) Induction of Alzheimer's disease type pathologies in cultured hippocampal slices by cholesterol depletion. Soc Neurosci 27: Abstr 963.17

Blaton V, Howard AN, Gresham GA, Vandamme D, Peeters H (1970) Lipid changes in the plasma lipoproteins of baboons given an atherogenic diet. I. Changes in the lipids of total plasma and of alpha and beta-lipoproteins. Atherosclerosis 11: 497–507

Blaton V, Vandamme D, Peeters H (1972) Chimpanzees and baboons as biochemical models for human atherosclerosis. Medical primatology. Basel: Karger; Proc 3rd Conf Exp Med Surg Primates, Lyon, part III: 306–312

Blaton V, Vandamme D, Declercq B, Vastesaeger M, Mortelmans J, Peeters H (1974 a) Dietary induced hyperbetalipoproteinemia in chimpanzees: comparison to the human hyperlipoproteinemia. Exp Mol Pathol 20: 132–146

Blaton V, Vercaemst R, Vandecasteele N, Caster H, Peeters H (1974 b) Isolation and partial characterization of chimpanzee plasma high density lipoproteins and their apolipoproteins. Biochemistry 13: 1127–1135

Blumenschine RJ (1987) Characteristics of an early hominid scavenging niche. Curr Anthropol 28: 383–407

Boerwinkle E, Leffert CC, Lin J, Lackner C, Chiesa G, Hobbs HH (1992) Apolipoprotein (a) gene accounts for greater than 90 % of the variation in plasma lipoprotein (a) concentrations. J Clin Invest 90: 52–60

Boesch C, Boesch H (1989) Hunting behavior of wild chimpanzees in the Taï National Park. Am J Phys Anthropol 78: 547–573

Breslow JL (2000) Genetics of lipoprotein abnormalities associated with coronary artery disease susceptibility. Annu Rev Genet 34: 233–254

British Nutrition Foundation (1992) Task force on unsaturated fatty acids. London: Chapman and Hall

Brown CM, Eyster MV, Sullivan PM, Colton CM, Vitek MP (2001) Gender differences in apolipoprotein E isoform regulation of nitric oxide release. Soc Neurosci Abstr 27: 583.12

Bunn HT, Kroll EM (1986) Systematic butchery by Plio/Pleistocene hominids at Olduvai Gorge, Tanzania. Curr Anthropol 27: 431–452

Carter DB, Dunn E, McKinley DD, Stratman NC, Boyle TP, Kuiper SL, Oostveen JA, Weaver RJ, Boller JA, Gurney ME (2001) Human apolipoprotein E4 accelerates beta-amyloid deposition in APPsw transgenic mouse brain. Ann Neurol 50: 468–475

Cernáková L, Brown P, Goldfarb LG, Nagle J, Pettrone K, Rubenstein R, Dubnick M, Gibbs CJ Jr, Gajdusek DC (1994) Infectious amyloid precursor gene sequences in primates used for experimental transmission of human spongiform encephalopathy. Proc Natl Acad Sci USA 91: 12 159–12 162

Chapman J, Cervenakova L, Petersen RB, Lee HS, Estupinan J, Richardson S, Vnencak-Jones CL, Gajdusek DC, Korczyn AD, Brown P, Goldfarb LG (1998) APOE in non-Alzheimer amyloidoses: transmissible spongiform encephalopathies. Neurology 51: 548–553

Charlesworth B (1996) Evolution of senescence: Alzheimer's disease and evolution. Curr Biol 6: 20–22

Clarkson TB, Weingand KW, Kaplan JR, Adams MR (1987) Mechanisms of atherogenesis. Circulation 76: 120–128

Connor KE, Morgan DG, Good RA, Walker CL, Engelman RW, Gordon MN (2000) Effects of caloric restriction on amyloid pathology in transgenic mice expressing both amyloid precursor protein and presenilin-1 mutations. Soc Neurosci 26: 181.15

Cordain L, Goitshall RW, Eaton SB (1997) Evolutionary aspects of exercise. In: Simopolous AP, (ed) Nutrition and fitness: evolutionary aspects. children's health, programs and policies. World reviews of nutrition and diet. Basel: Karger 81: 49–60

Cordain L, Gotshall RW, Eaton BS, Eaton BS III (1998) Physical activity, energy expenditure, and fitness: an evolutionary perspective. Int J Sports Med 19: 328–335

Cordain L, Watkins BA, Mann N (2001) Fatty acid composition and energy density of foods available to African hominids. In: Simopolous AP, Pavlou KN (eds) Nutrition and fitness: metabolic studies in health and disease. World reviews of nutrition and diet. Basel: Karger 90: 144–161

Cordain L, Eaton SB, Miller JB, Mann N, Hill K (2002 a) The paradoxical nature of hunter-gatherer diets: meat-based, yet nonatherogenic. Eur J Clin Nutrit 56 (Supp 1) S 1–11

Cordain L, Watkins BA, Florant GL, Kelher M, Rogers L, Li Y (2002 b) Fatty acid analysis of wild ruminant tissues: evolutionary implications for reducing diet-related chronic disease. Eur J Clin Nutrit 56: 1–11

Corder EH, Robertson K, Lannfelt L, Bogdanovic N, Eggertsen G, Wilkins J, Hall C (1998) HIV-infected subjects with the E4 allele for APOE have excess dementia and peripheral neuropathy. Nat Med 4: 1182–1184

Courtenay J, Santow G (1989) Mortality of wild and captive chimpanzees. Folia Primatol 52: 167–177

Crawford MA (1992) The role of dietary fatty acids in biology: their place in the evolution of the human brain. Nutr Rev 50: 3–11

Danner DD, Snowdon DA, Friesen WV (2001) Positive emotions in early life and longevity: findings from the nun study. J Pers Soc Psychol 80: 804–813

Dart R (1953) The predatory transition from ape to man. Int Anthropol Linguistic Rev 1: 201–219

Defleur A, White T, Valensi P, Slimak L, Cregut-Bonnoure E (1999) Neanderthal cannibalism at Moula-Guercy, Ardeche, France. Science 286: 128–131

Deschamps V, Barberger-Gateau P, Peuchant E, Orgogozo JM (2001) Nutritional factors in cerebral aging and dementia: epidemiological arguments for a role of oxidative stress. Neuroepidemiology 20: 7–15

Distl R, Meske V, Ohm TG (2001) Tangle-bearing neurons contains more free cholesterol than adjacent tangle free neurons. Acta Neuropathol 101: 547–554

Dock W (1971) Fat metabolism in the Masai. N Engl J Med 285: 58–59

Doucet C, Huby T, Chapman J, Thillet J (1994) Lipoprotein (a) in the chimpanzee: relationship of apo (a) phenotype to elevated plasma Lp (a) levels. J Lipids Res 35: 263–270

Eaton SB, Eaton SB III, Sinclair AJ, Cordain L, Munn NJ (1998) Dietary intake of long-chain polyunsaturated fatty acids during the paleolithic. In: Simopolous AP (ed) The return of omega-3 fatty acids into the food supply. Land-based animal food products and their health effects. World reviews of nutrition and diet. Basel: Karger 83: 12–23

Evans RM, Emsley CL, Gao S, Sahota A, Hall KS, Farlow MR, Hendrie H (2000) Serum cholesterol, ApoE genotype, and the risk of Alzheimer's disease: a population-based study of African Americans. Neurology 54: 240–242

Fan QW, Yu W, Senda T, Yanagisawa K, Michikawa M (2001) Cholesterol-dependent modulation of tau phosphorylation in cultured neurons. J Neurochem 76: 391–400

Farrer LA, Cupples LA, Haines JL, Hyman B, Kukull WA, Mayeux R, Myers RH, Pericak-Vance MA, Risch N, van Duijn CM (1997) Effects of age, sex, and ethnicity on the association between apolipoprotein E genotype and Alzheimer disease. A meta-analysis APOE and Alzheimer Disease Meta Analysis Consortium. J Am Med Assoc 278: 1349–1355

Fassbender K, Simons M, Bergmann C, Stroick M, Lutjohann D, Keller P, Runz H, Kuhl S, Bertsch T, von Bergmann K, Hennerici M, Beyreuther K, Hartmann T (2001) Simvastatin strongly reduces levels of Alzheimer's disease beta-amyloid peptides Abeta 42 and Abeta 40 in vitro and in vivo. Proc Natl Acad Sci USA 98: 5856–5861

Finch CE (1990) Longevity, senescence, and the genome. Chicago: U Chicago Press

Finch CE (2002) Evolution and the plasticity of aging in the reproductive schedules in long-lived animals: the importance of genetic variation in neuroendocrine mechanisms. In: Pfaff D, Arnold A, Etgen A, Fahrbach S, Rubin R (eds) Hormones, brain, and behavior. San Diego: Academic Press, vol 4: 799–820

Finch CE, Sapolsky RM (1999) The evolution of Alzheimer disease, the reproductive schedule, and apoE isoforms. Neurobiol Aging 20: 407–428

Finch CE, Kirkwood TBL (2000) Chance, development, and aging. Oxford: Oxford University Press

Finch CE, Longo V (2000) The gero-inflammatory manifold. In: Rogers J (ed) Neuroinflammatory mechanisms in Alzheimer's disease: basic and clinical research. Basel: Birkhäuser Verlag

Finch CE, Pike MC, Witten M (1990) Slow mortality rate accelerations during aging in some animals approximate that of humans. Science 249: 902–905

Forslund AH, Hambraeus L, Olsson RM, El-Khoury AE, Yu YM, Young VR (1998) The 24-h whole body leucine and urea kinetics at normal and high protein intakes with exercise in healthy adults. Am J Physiol 275: E 310–320

Forslund AH, El-Khoury AE, Olsson RM, Sjodin AM, Hambraeus L, Young VR (1999) Effect of protein intake and physical activity on 24-h pattern and rate of macronutrient utilization. Am J Physiol 276: E 964–976

Friedland RP, Fritsch T, Smyth KA, Koss E, Lerner AJ, Chen CH, Petot GJ, Debanne SM (2001) Patients with Alzheimer's disease have reduced activities in midlife compared with healthy control-group members. Proc Natl Acad Sci USA 98: 3440–3445

Fullerton SM, Clark AG, Weiss KM, Nickerson DA, Taylor SL, Stengard JH, Salomaa V, Vartiainen E, Perola M, Boerwinkle E, Sing CF (2000) Apolipoprotein E variation at the sequence haplotype level: implications for the origin and maintenance of a major human polymorphism. Am J Human Genet 67: 881–900

Gagneux P, Varki A (2001) Genetic difference between humans and great apes. Mol Phylogenet Evol 18: 2–13

Gagneux P, Gonder MK, Goldberg TL, Morin PA (2001) Gene flow in wild chimpanzee populations: what genetic data tell us about chimpanzee movement over space and time. Philos Trans R Soc Lond B Biol Sci 356: 889–897

Gearing M, Rebeck GW, Hyman BT, Tigges J, Mirra SS (1994) Neuropathology and apolipoprotein E profile of aged chimpanzees: implications for Alzheimer disease. Proc Natl Acad Sci USA 91: 9382–9386

Gearing M, Tigges J, Mori H, Mirra SS (1996) A beta40 ist a major form of beta-amyloid in nonhuman primates. Neurobiol Aging 17: 903–908

Gearing M, Tigges J, Mori H, Mirra SS (1997) beta-Amyloid (A beta) deposition in the brains of aged orangutans. Neurobiol Aging 18: 139–146

Gerdes LU, Gerdes C, Hansen PS, Klausen IC, Faergeman O (1996) Are men carrying the apolipoprotein epsilon 4- or epsilon 2 allele less fertile than epsilon 3 epsilon 3 genotypes? Human Genet 98: 239–242

Gomez-Isla T, Price JL, McKeel DW Jr, Morris JC, Growdon JH, Hyman BT (1996) Profound loss of layer II entorhinal cortex neurons occurs in very mild Alzheimer's disease. J Neurosci 16: 4491–5000

Goodall J (1983) Population dynamics during a fifteen-year period in one commnity of free-living chimpanzees in the Gombe National Park, Tanzania. Zeitschr Tierpsychol 61: 1–60

Goodall J (1986) The chimpanzees of the Gombe. Patterns of behavior. Cambridge: Cambridge University Press

Hagberg JM, Wilund KR, Ferrell RE (2000) ApoE gene and gene environment effects on plasma lipoprotein-lipid levels. Physiol Genomics 4: 101–108

Hanlon CS, Rubinsztein DC (1995) Arginine residues at codons 112 and 158 in the apolipoprotein E gene correspond to the ancestral state in humans. Arthrosclerosis 112: 85–90

Härtig W, Bruckner G, Schmidt C, Brauer K, Bodewitz G, Turner JD, Bigl V (1997) Co-localization of beta-amyloid peptides, apolipoprotein E and glial markers in senile plaques in the prefrontal cortex of old rhesus monkeys. Brain Res 751: 315–322

Härtig W, Klein C, Brauer K, Schuppel KF, Arendt T, Bruckner G, Bigl V (2000) Abnormally phosphorylated protein tau in the cortex of aged individuals of various mammalian orders. Acta Neuropathol (Berl). 100: 305–312

Hartmann RE, Wozniak DF, Nardi A, Olney JW, Sartorius L, Holtzman DM (2001) Behavioral phenotyping of GFAP-apoE3 and -apoE4 transgenic mice: apoE4 mice show profound working memory impairments in the absence of Alzheimer's-like neuropatholog. Exp

Hendrie HC, Ogunniyi A, Hall KS, Baiyewu O, Unverzagt FW, Gureje O, Gao S, Evans RM, Ogunseyinde AO, Adeyinka AO, Musick B, Hui SL (2001) Incidence of dementia and Alzheimer disease in 2 communities: Yoruba residing in Ibadan, Nigeria, and African Americans residing in Indianapolis, Indiana. J Am Med Assoc 285: 739–747

Hill K, Boesch C, Goodall J, Pusey A, Williams J, Wrangham R (2001) Mortality rates among wild chimpanzees. J Human Evol 40: 437–450

Horai S, Satta Y, Hayasaka K, Kondo R, Inoue T, Ishida T, Hayashi S, Takahata N (1992) Man's place in Hominoidea revealed by mitochondrial DNA geneology. J Mol Evol 35: 32–43

Holtzman DM, Bales KR, Tenkova T, Fagan AM, Parsadanian M, Sartorius LJ, Mackey B, Olney J, McKeel D, Wozniak D, Paul SM (2000) Apolipoprotein E isoform-dependent amyloid deposition and neuritic degeneration in a mouse model of Alzheimer's disease. Proc Natl Acad Sci USA 97: 2892–2897

Howard AN, Blaton V, Vandamme D, Van Landschoot N, Peeters H (1972) Lipid changes in the plasma lipoproteins of baboons given an atherogenic diet. 3. A comparison between lipid changes in the plasma of the baboon and chimpanzee given atherogenic diets and those in human plasma lipoproteins of type II hyperlipoproteinaemia. Atherosclerosis 16: 257–272

Hu J, LaDu MJ, Van Eldik LJ (1998) Apolipoprotein E attenuates beta-amyloid-induced astrocyte activation. J Neurochem 71: 1626–1634

Huang Y, Liu XQ, Wyss-Coray T, Brecht WJ, Sanan DA, Mahley RW (2001) Apolipoprotein E fragments present in Alzheimer's disease brains induce neurofibrillary tangle-like intracellular inclusions in neurons. Proc Natl Acad Sci USA 98: 8838–8843

Huby T, Dachet C, Lawn RM, Wickings J, Chapman MJ, Tillet J (2001) Functional analysis of the chimpanzee and human apo (a) promoter sequences: identification of sequence variations responsible for elevated transcriptional activity in chimpanzee. J Biol Chem 276: 22 209–22 214

Innes S (2000) The role of dietary n-6 and n-3 fatty acids in the developing brain. Dev Neurosci 22: 474–480

Isaac GL, Crader DC (1981) To what extent were early hominids carnivorous? An archaeological perspective. In: Harding RSO, Teleki G (eds) Omnivorous primates. New York: Columbia University Press, pp 37–103

Jick H, Zornberg GL, Jick SS, Seshadri S, Drachman DA (2000) Statins and the risk of dementia. Lancet 356: 1627–1631

Kalmijn S (2000) Fatty acid intake and the risk of dementia and cognitive decline: a review of clinical and epidemiological studies. J Nutr Health Aging 4: 202–207

Kaplan HS, Hill K, Lancaster J, Hurtado AM (2001) A theory of human life history evolution: diet, intelligence, and longevity. Evol Anthropol 9: 156–184

Kivipelto M, Helkala EL, Laakso MP, Hanninen T, Hallikainen M, Alhainen K, Soininen H, Tuomilehto J, Nissinen A (2001) Midlife vascular risk factors and Alzheimer's disease in later life: longitudinal, population based study. Brit Med J 322: 1447–1451

Klein WL, Krafft GA, Finch CE (2001) Targeting small Aβ oligomers: the solution to an Alzheimer's disease conundrum? Trends Neurosci 24: 219–224

Kojro E, Gimpl G, Lammich S, Marz W, Fahrenholz F (2001) Low cholesterol stimulates the nonamyloidogenic pathway by its effect on the alpha-secretase ADAM 10. Proc Natl Acad Sci USA 98: 5815–5820

Korte W, Greiner J, Feldges A, Riesen WF (2001) Increased lipoprotein (a) levels are a steady prothrombotic defect. Blood 98: 1993–1994

Koudinov AR, Berezov TT, Koudinova NV (2001) The levels of soluble amyloid beta indifferent high density lipoprotein sub fractions distinguish Alzheimer's and normal aging cerebrospinal fluid: implication fn brain cholesterol pathology. Neurosci Let 314: 115–118

Lambert MP, Barlow AK, Chromy B, Edwards C, Freed R, Liosatos M, Morgan TE, Rozovsky I, Trommer B, Viola KL, Wals P, Zhang C, Finch CE, Krafft GA, Klein WL (1998) Diffusible, non-fibrillar ligands derived from Aβ1–42. Proc Natl Acad Sci USA 95: 6448–6453

Lambert MP, Viola KL, Chromy BA, Chang L, Morgan TE, Yu J, Venton DL, Krafft GA, Finch CE, Klein WL (2001) Vaccination with soluble Aβ oligomers generates toxicity-neutralizing antibodies. J Neurochem 79: 595–605

Leistikow EA (1998) Is coronary artery disease initiated perinatally? Semin Thromb Hemost 24: 139–143

Liberski PP, Gajdusek DC (1997) Kuru: forty years later, a historical note. Brain Pathol 7: 555–760

Lindsay S, Chaikoff IL (1966) Naturally occurring arteriosclerosis in nonhuman primates. J Atheroscler Res 6: 36–61

Mahley RW, Rall Jr SC (2000) Apolipoprotein E: far more than a lipid transport protein. Ann Rev Genomics Hum Genet 1: 507–537

Mann GV (1964) Cardiovascular disease in the Masai. Atheroscler Res 4: 289–312

Mann GV (1972) Sterol metabolism in the chimpanzee. Medical primatology. Basel: Karger, Proc 3rd Conf Exp Med Surg Primates, Lyon, part III: 324–325

Mann GV, Shaffer RD (1966) Cholesteremia in pregnant Masai women. J Am Med Assoc 197: 1071–1073

Mann GV, Shaffer RD, Rich A (1965) Physical fitness and immunity to heart-disease in Masai. Lancet 2 (7426): 1308–1310

Mann GV, McNamara JJ, Macomber PB, Wroblewski R (1971) Coronary artery disease in Vietnam casualties. J Am Med Assoc 217: 478–479

Mann GV, Spoerry A, Gray M, Jarashow D (1972) Atherosclerosis in the Masai. Am J Epidemiol 95: 26–37

Manning GW (1942) Coronary disease in the ape. Am Heart J 23: 719–724

Martin GM (1999) APOE alleles and lipophylic pathogens. Neurobiol Aging 20: 441–443

Marx J (2001) Bad for the heart, bad for the mind? Science 294: 508–509

Mattila KJ, Asikainen S, Wolf J, Jousimies-Somer H, Valtonen V, Nieminen M (2000) Age, dental infections, and coronary heart disease. J Dent Res 79: 756–760

Mayeux R, Costa R, Bell K, Merchant C, Tang MX, Jacobs D (1999) Reduced risk of Alzheimer's disease among individuals with low calorie intake. Am Acad Neurol 52 (Suppl 2): A296–A297

McGeer PL, Walker DG, Pitas RE, Mahley RW, McGeer EG (1997) Apolipoprotein E4 (ApoE4) but not ApoE3 or ApoE2 potentiates beta-amyloid protein activation of complement in vitro. Brain Res 749: 135–138

McGrew WC (1992) Chimpanzee material culture. Cambridge University Press, Cambridge

Merrill DA, Chiba AA, Tuszynski MH (2001) Conservation of neuronal number and size in the entorhinal cortex of behaviorally characterized aged rats. J Comp Neurol 438: 445–456

Mills J, Reiner PB (1999) Regulation of amyloid precursor protein cleavage. J Neurochem 72: 443–460

Milton K (1999) A hypothesis to explain the role of meat-eating in human evolution. Evol Anthropol 8: 11–21

Moir RD, Atwood CS, Romano DM, Laurans MH, Huang X, Bush AI, Smith JD, Tanzi RE (1999) Differential effects of apolipoprotein E isoforms on metal-induced aggregation of A beta using physiological concentrations. Biochemistry 38: 4595–4603

Montine KS, Olson SJ, Amarnath V, Whetsell WO Jr, Graham DG, Montine TJ (1997) Immunohistochemical detection of 4-hydroxy-2-nonenal adducts in Alzheimer's disease is associated with inheritance of APOE4. Am J Pathol 150: 437–443

Moore SA (2001) Polyunsaturated fatty acid synthesis and release by brain-derived cells in vitro. J Mol Neurosci 16: 195–200

Morrell P, Quarles RH (1999) Myelin formation, structure, and biochemistry. In: Siegel G, Agranoff BW, Uhler ME (eds) Basic neurochemistry: molecular, cellular, and medical aspects. 6th ed. Philadelphia: Lippincott-Raven, pp. 70–92

Mucke L, Masliah E, Yu GQ, Mallory M, Rockenstein EM, Tatsuno G, Hu K, Kholodenko D, Johnson-Wood K, McConlogue L (2000) High-level neuronal expression of abeta 1–42 in wild-type human amyloid protein precursor transgenic mice: synaptotoxicity without plaque formation. J Neurosci 20: 4050–4058

Nakagawa Y, Kitamoto T, Furukawa H, Ogomori K, Tateishi J (1995) Allelic variation of apolipoprotein E in Japanese sporadic Creutzfeldt-Jakob disease patients. Neurosci Lett 187: 209–211

Nelson CA, Greer WE, Morris MD (1984) The distribution of serum high density lipoprotein subfractions in non-human primates. Lipid 19: 656–663

Newman PE (1998) Could diet be used to reduce the risk of developing Alzheimer's disease? Med Hypotheses 50: 335–337

Normile D (2001) Comparative genomics. Gene expression differs in human and chimp brains. Science 292: 44–45

Notkola IL, Sulkava R, Pekkanen J, Erkinjuntti T, Ehnholm C, Kivinen P, Tuomilehto J, Nissinen A (1998) Serum total cholesterol, apolipoprotein E epsilon 4 allele, and Alzheimer's disease. Neuroepidemiology 17: 14–20

Nowak RM, Paradiso JL (1983) Walker's mammals of the world. 2 Vols. Baltimore: Johns Hopkins University Press

Oda T, Wals P, Osterburg HH, Johnson SA, Pasinetti GM, Morgan TE, Rozovsky I, Stine WB, Snyder SW, Holzman TF, Krafft GA, Finch CE (1995) Clusterin (apoJ) alters the aggregation of amyloid β-peptide (Aβ1–42) and forms slowly sedimenting Aβ complexes that cause oxidative stress. Exp Neurol 136: 22–31

Patel NC, Finch CE (2002) The glucocorticoid paradox of caloric restriction in slowing brain aging. Neurobiol Aging, in press

Peeters H, Blaton V (1972) Comparative lipid values of human and nonhuman primates. Medical primatology. Basel: Karger, Proc 3rd Conf Exp Med Surg Primates, Lyon, part III: 336–342

Peeters H, Blaton V, Declercq B, Howard AN, Gresham GA (1970) Lipid changes in the plasma lipoproteins of baboons given an atherogenic diet, 2. Changes in the phospholipid classes of total plasma and of alpha- and beta-lipoproteins. Atherosclerosis 12: 283–290

Peng DQ, Zhao SP, Wang JL (1999) Lipoprotein (a) and apolipoprotein E epsilon 4 as independent risk factors for ischemic stroke. J Cardiovasc Risk 6: 1–6

Pickering-Brown SM, Mann DM, Owen F, Ironside JW, de Silva R, Roberts DA, Balderson DJ, Cooper PN (1995) Allelic variations in apolipoprotein E and prion protein genotype related to plaque formation and age of onset in sporadic Creutzfeldt-Jakob disease. Neurosci Lett 187: 127–129

Planas J, Grau M (1971) Serum chemistry in the chimpanzee and the gorilla. Folia Primatol 15: 77–87

Poirier J (2000) Apolipoprotein E and Alzheimer's disease. A role in amyloid catabolism. Ann NY Acad Sci 924: 81–90

Price DL, Martin LJ, Sisodia SS, Wagster MV, Koo EH, Walker LC, Koliatsos VE, Cork LC (1991) Aged non-human primates: an animal model of age-associated neurodegenerative disease. Brain Pathol 1: 287–296

Prusiner SB, Hsiao KK (1994) Human prion diseases. Ann Neurol 35: 385–395

Prusiner SB, Safar J, Cohen FE, DeArmond SJ (1999) The prion diseases. In: Terry RD, Katzman R, Bick KL, Sisodia SS (eds) Alzheimer disease. 2nd Ed. Lippencott Williams and Wilkins, Philadelphia, pp. 161–179

Puglielli L, Konopka G, Pack-Chung E, Ingano LA, Berezovska O, Hyman BT, Chang TY, Tanzi RE, Kovacs DM (2001) Acyl-coenzyme A: cholesterol acyltransferase modulates the generation of the amyloid beta-peptide. Nat Cell Biol 3: 905–912

Ramassamy C, Averill D, Beffert U, Bastianetto S, Theroux L, Lussier-Cacan S, Cohn JS, Christen Y, Davignon J, Quirion R, Poirier J (1999) Oxidative damage and protection by antioxidants in the frontal cortex of Alzheimer's disease is related to the apolipoprotein E genotype. Free Radic Biol Med 27: 544–553

Rasmussen T, Schliemann T, Sorensen JC, Zimmer J, West MJ (1996) Memory impaired aged rats: no loss of principal hippocampal and subicular neurons. Neurobiol Aging 17: 143–147

Ratcliffe HL (1965) Age and environment as factors in the nature and frequency of cardiovascular lesions in mammals and bird in the Philadelphia zoological garden. Ann NY Acad Sci 127: 715–735

Ravnskov U (1998) The questionable role of saturated and polyunsaturated fatty acids in cardiovascular disease. J Clin Epidemiol 51: 443–460

Refolo LM, Malester B, LaFrancois J, Bryant-Thomas T, Wang R, Tint GS, Sambamurti K, Duff K, Pappolla MA (2000) Hypercholesterolemia accelerates the Alzheimer's amyloid pathology in a transgenic mouse model. Neurobiol Dis 7: 321–331

Reiman EM, Caselli RJ, Yun LS, Chen K, Bandy D, Minoshima S, Thibodeau SN, Osborne D (1996) Preclinical evidence of Alzheimer's disease in persons homozygous for the epsilon 4 allele for apolipoprotein E. N Engl J Med 334: 752–758

Riddell DR, Christie G, Hussain I, Dingwall C (2001) Compartmentalization of beta-secretase (Asp2) into low-buoyant density, noncaveolar lipid rafts. Curr Biol 11: 1288–1293

Roses AD (1998) Alzheimer diseases: a model of gene mutations and susceptibility polymorphisms for complex psychiatric diseases. Am J Med Genet 81: 49–57

Rosseneu M, Declercq B, Vandamme D, Vercaemst R, Soetewey F, Peeters H, Blaton V (1979) Influence of oral polyunsaturated and saturated phospholipid treatment on the lipid composition and fatty acid profile of chimpanzee lipoproteins. Atherosclerosis 32: 141–153

Rudman D, DiFulco TJ, Galambos JT, Smith RB 3rd, Salam AA, Warren WD (1973) Maximal rates of excretion and synthesis of urea in normal and cirrhotic subjects. J Clin Invest 52: 2241–2249

Ruvolo M, Disotell TR, Allard MW, Brown WM, Honeycutt RL (1991) Resolution of the African hominoid trichotomy by use of a mitochondrial gene sequence. Proc Natl Acad Sci USA 88: 1570–1574

Salvatore M, Seeber AC, Nacmias B, Petraroli R, D'Alessandro M, Sorbi S, Pocchiari M (1995) Apolipoprotein E in sporadic and familial Creutzfeldt-Jakob disease. Neurosci Lett 199: 95–98

Sammon AM (1999) Dietary linoleic acid, immune inhibition and disease. Postgrad Med 75: 129–132

Sanders TA (1999) Essential fatty acid requirements of vegetarians in pregnancy, lactation, and infancy. Am J Clin Nutr 70 (3 Suppl): 555S–559S

Sapolsky RM, Mott GE (1987) Social subordinance in wild baboons is associated with suppressed high density lipoprotein-cholesterol concentrations: the possible role of chronic social stress. Endocrinology 121: 1605–1610

Sawamura N, Gong JS, Gauer WS, Heidenreich RA, Ninomiya H, Ohno K, Yanagisawa K, Michikawa M (2001) Site specific phosphorylation of tau accompagnied by activation of mitogen-activated protein kinase (MAPK) in brains of Niemann-Pick type C mice. J Biol Chem 276: 10 314–10 319

Schätzl HM, Da Costa M, Taylor L, Cohen FE, Prusiner SB (1995) Prion protein gene variation among primates. J Mol Biol 245: 362–374; erratum in J Mol Biol (1997) Jan 17; 265 (2): 257

Schmidt R (1978) Systematic pathology of chimpanzees. J Med Primatol 7: 274–318

Selkoe DJ, Bell DS, Podlisny MB, Price DL, Cork LC (1987) Conservation of brain amyloid proteins in aged mammals and humans with Alzheimer's disease. Science 235: 873–877

Severinghaus CW (1949) Tooth development and wear as criteria of age in white-tailed deer. J Wildlife Mgt 13: 195–216

Sharp PM, Bailes E, Chaudhuri RR, Rodenburg CM, Santiago MO, Hahn BH (2001) The origins of acquired immune deficiency syndrome viruses: where and when? Philos Trans Roy Soc Lond B Biol Sci 356: 867–876

Sharrett AR, Ballantyne CM, Coady SA, Heiss G, Sorlie PD, Catellier D, Patsch W (2001) Coronary heart disease prediction from lipoprotein cholesterol levels, triglycerides, lipoprotein (a), apolipoproteins A-I and B, and HDL density subfractions: the atherosclerosis risk in communities (ARIC) study. Circulation 104: 1108–1113

Shipman P (1986) Scavenging or hunting in early hominids: theoretical framework and tests. Am Anthropol 88: 27–43

Sikes SK (1971) The natural history of the African elephant. New York: American Elsevier

Simons M, Keller P, Dichgans J, Schulz JB (2001) Cholesterol and Alzheimer's disease: is there a link? Neurology 57: 1089–1093

Small GW, Ercoli LM, Silverman DH, Huang SC, Komo S, Bookheimer SY, Lavretsky H, Miller K, Siddarth P, Rasgon NL, Mazziotta JC, Saxena S, Wu HM, Mega MS, Cummings JL, Saunders AM, Pericak-Vance MA, Roses AD, Barrio JR, Phelps M (2000) Cerebral metabolic and cognitive decline in persons at genetic risk for Alzheimer's disease. Proc Natl Acad Sci USA 97: 6037–6042

Snowdon DA, Kemper SJ, Mortimer JA, Greiner LH, Wekstein DR, Markesbery WR (1996) Linguistic ability in early life and cognitive function and Alzheimer's disease in late life. Findings from the Nun Study. J Am Med Assoc 275: 528–532

Sohal RS, Weindruch R (1996) Oxidative stress, caloric restriction, and aging. Science 273: 59–63

Sparks DL (1996) Intraneuronal beta-amyloid immunoreactivity in the CNS. Neurobiol Aging 17: 291–299

Speth JD (1989) Early hominid hunting and scavenging: the role of meat as an enery source. J Human Evol 18: 329–343

Speth JD (1991) Protein selection and avoidance strategies of contemporary and ancestral forages: unresolved issues. Phil Trans Roy Soc London, Series B: 334: 265–270

Speth JD, Tchernov E (2001) Neandertal hunting and meat-processing in the Near East: evidence from Kebara Cave (Israel). In: Stanford CB, Bunn HT (eds) Meat-eating and human evolution. Oxford: Oxford U. Press, pp. 52–72

Srinivasan SR, McBride JR Jr, Radhakrishnamurthy B, Berenson GS (1974) Comparative studies of serum lipoprotein and lipid profiles in subhuman primates. Comp Biochem Physiol B 47: 711–716

Srinivasan S, Radhakrishnamurthy B, Dalferes E, Berenson G (1979) Serum alpha-lipoprotein responses to variations in dietary cholesterol, protein and carbohydrate in different non-human primate species. Lipids 14: 559–565

Stanford CB (1998) Chimpanzee and red colobus. Cambridge MA: Harvard University Press

Stanford CB (1999) The hunting apes. Princeton: Princeton University Press

Stanford CB, Bunn HT (2001) Meat-eating and human evolution. Oxford: Oxford University Press

Stanford CB, Wallis J, Matama H, Goodallt J (1994) Patterns of predation by chimpanzees on red colobus monkeys in Gombe National Park, 1982–1991. Am J Phys Antropol 94: 213–228

Steinetz BG, Randolph C, Cohn D, Mahoney CJ (1996) Lipoprotein profiles and glucose tolerance in lean and obese chimpanzees. J Med Primatol 25: 17–25

Stewart R, Russ C, Richards M, Brayne C, Lovestone S, Mann A (2001) Apolipoprotein E genotype, vascular risk and early cognitive impairment in an African Caribbean population. Dement Geriatr Cogn Disord 12: 251–256

Stiner MC (2001) Carnivory, coevolution, and the geographic spread of the genus Homo. J Archaeol Res, in press

Strong JP, Eggen DA, Newman III WP, Martinez RD (1968) Naturally occurring and experimental atherosclerosis in primates. Ann NY Acad Sci 149: 882–894

Tang MX, Stern Y, Marder K, Bell K, Gurland B, Lantigua R, Andrews H, Feng L, Tycko B, Mayeux R (1998) The APOE-epsilon 4 allele and the risk of Alzheimer disease among African Americans, whites, and Hispanics. J Am Med Assoc 279: 751–755

Taylor DM (1999) Inactivation of prions by physical and chemical means. J Hosp Infect 43: S69–S76

Telling GC, Haga T, Torchia M, Tremblay P, DeArmond SJ, Prusiner SB (1996) Interactions between wild-type and mutant prion proteins modulate neurodegeneration in transgenic mice. Genes Dev 10: 1736–1750

Thomas H (1997) The slave trade: the story of the Atlantic slave trade 1440–1870. Boston: Simon & Schuster

Tikkanen M, Huttunen JK, Pajukanta PE, Pietinen P (1995) Apolipoprotein E polymorphism and dietary plasma cholesterol response. Can J Cardiol Suppl G: 93G–96G

Ungar PS, Kay RF (1995) The dietary adaptations of European Miocene catarrhines. Proc Natl Acad Sci USA 92: 5479–5481

Van Liew JB, Davis PJ, Davis FB, Bernardis LL, Deziel MR, Marinucci LN, Kumar D (1993) Effects of aging, diet, and sex on plasma glucose, fructosamine, and lipid concentrations in barrier-raised Fischer 344 rats. J Gerontol 48: B184–190

Vastesaeger MM, Vercruysse J, Martin JJ (1972) Pitfalls of experimental atherosclerosis in the chimpanzee. Medical Primatology. Basel: Karger; Proc 3rd Conf Exp Med Surg Primates, Lyon, part III: 376–381

Vaupel JW, Carey JR, Christensen K, Johnson TE, Yashin AI, Holm NV, Iachine IA, Kannisto V, Khazaeli AA, Liedo P, Longo VD, Zeng Y, Manton KG, Curtsinger JW (1998) Biodemographic trajectories of longevity. Science 280: 855–860

West MJ, Coleman PD, Flood DG, Troncoso JC (1994) Differences in the pattern of hippocampal neuronal loss in normal ageing and Alzheimer's disease. Lancet 344: 769–772

Williard DE, Harmon SD, Kaduce TL, Preuss M, Moore SA, Robbins ME, Spector AA (2001) Docosahexaenoic acid synthesis from n-3 polyunsaturated fatty acids in differentiated rat brain astrocytes. J Lipid Res 42: 1368–1376

Wissler RW, Vesselinovitch D (1968) Comparative pathogenetic patterns in atherosclerosis. Adv Lipid Res 6: 181–206

Wolozin B (2001) A fluid connection: cholesterol and Abeta. Proc Natl Acad Sci USA 98: 5371–5373

Wolozin B, Kellman W, Ruosseau P, Celesia GG, Siegel G (2000) Decreased prevalence of Alzheimer disease associated with 3-hydroxy, 4-methyglutaryl coenzyme A reductase inhibitors. Arch Neurol 57: 1439–1443

Woodruff-Pak DS, Steinmetz JE, Thompson RF (1988) Classical conditioning of rabbits $2^{1}/_{2}$ to 4 years old using mossy fiber stimulation as a CS. Neurobiol Aging 9: 187–193

Wrangham RW (1975) Behavioural ecology of chimpanzees in Gombe National Park, Tanzania. PhD dissertation, University of Cambridge

Xu Q, Li Y, Cyras C, Sanan DA, Cordell B (2000) Isolation and characterization of apolipoproteins from murine microglia identification of a low density lipoprotein-like apolipoprotein J-rich but E-poor spherical particle. J Biol Chem 275: 31 770–31 777

Yanagisawa M, Planel E, Ishiguro K, Fujita SC (1999) Starvation induces tau hyperphosphorylation in mouse brain: implications for Alzheimer's disease. FEBS Lett 461: 329–333

Yip CM, Elton EA, Darabie AA, Morrison MR, McLaurin J (2001) Cholesterol, a modulator of membrane-associated Abeta-fibrillogenesis and neurotoxicity. J Mol Biol 311: 723–734

Zarazaga A, Garcia-De-Lorenzo L, Garcia-Luna PP, Garcia-Peris P, Lopez-Martinez J, Lorenzo V, Quecedo L, Del Llano J (2001) Nutritional support in chronic renal failure: systematic review. Clin Nutr 20: 291–299

Zerr I, Helmhold M, Poser S, Armstrong VW, Weber T (1996) Apolipoprotein E phenotype frequency and cerebrospinal fluid concentration are not associated with Creutzfeldt-Jakob disease. Arch Neurol 53: 1233–1238

Zihlman AL, Morbeck ME, Sumner DR (1989) Tales of Gombe chimps as told in their bones. Anthroquest (Leakey Foundation News) 40: 20–22

Neural Capital and Life span Evolution among Primates and Humans

H. S. Kaplan, T. Mueller, S. Gangestad, J. B. Lancaster

Introduction

This paper presents a theory of brain and life span evolution and applies it to both the primate order, in general, and to the hominid line, in particular. To address the simultaneous effects of natural selection on the brain and on the life span, it extends standard life history theory (LHT) in biology, which organizes research into the evolutionary forces shaping age-schedules of fertility and mortality (Cole 1954; Gadgil and Bossert 1970; Partridge and Harvey 1985). This extension, *the embodied capital theory* (Kaplan and Robson 2001 b; Kaplan 1997; Kaplan et al. 2000), integrates existing models with an economic analysis of capital investments and the value of life.

The chapter begins with a brief introduction to embodied capital theory and then applies it to understanding major trends in primate evolution and the specific characteristics of humans. The evolution of brain size, intelligence and life histories in the primate order are addressed first. The evolution of human life course is then considered, with a specific focus on the relationship between cognitive development, economic productivity and longevity. It will be argued that the evolution of the human brain entailed a series of co-evolutionary responses in human development and aging, resulting in a highly structured species-typical life span that can vary within a limited range.

The Embodied Capital Theory of Life History Evolution

According to the theory of evolution by natural selection, the evolution of life is the result of a process in which variant forms compete to harvest energy from the environment and convert that energy into replicates of those forms. Those forms that can capture more energy than others and can convert the energy they acquire more efficiently into replicates than others become more prevalent through time. This simple issue of harvesting energy and converting energy into offspring generates many complex problems that are time-dependent.

Two fundamental tradeoffs determine the action of natural selection on reproductive schedules and mortality rates. The first tradeoff is between current and future reproduction. By growing, an organism can increase its energy capture rates in the future and thus increase its future fertility. For this reason,

Finch et al. (Eds.)
Brain and Longevity
© Springer-Verlag Berlin Heidelberg 2003

organisms typically have a juvenile phase in which fertility is zero until they reach a size at which some allocation to reproduction increases lifetime fitness more than growth. Similarly, among organisms that engage in repeated bouts of reproduction (humans included), some energy during the reproductive phase is diverted away from reproduction and allocated to maintenance so that they can live to reproduce again. Natural selection is expected to optimize the allocation of energy to current reproduction and to future reproduction (via investments in growth and maintenance) at each point in the life course so that genetic descendents are maximized (Gadgil and Bossert 1970). Variation across taxa and across conditions in optimal energy allocations is shaped by ecological factors, such as food supply, disease and predation rates.

A second fundamental life history tradeoff is between offspring number (quantity) and offspring fitness (quality). This tradeoff occurs because parents have limited resources to invest in offspring and each additional offspring produced necessarily reduces average investment per offspring. Most biological models (Lack 1954; Lloyd 1987; Smith and Fretwell 1974) operationalize this tradeoff as number vs. survival of offspring. However, parental investment may affect not only survival to adulthood but also the adult productivity and fertility of offspring. This is especially true of humans. Thus, natural selection is expected to shape investment per offspring and offspring number so as to maximize offspring number times their average lifetime fitness.

The embodied capital theory generalizes existing LHT by treating the processes of growth, development and maintenance as investments in stocks of somatic or embodied capital. In a physical sense, embodied capital is organized somatic tissue – muscles, digestive organs, brains, etc. In a functional sense, embodied capital includes strength, speed, immune function, skill, knowledge and other abilities. Since such stocks tend to depreciate with time, allocations to maintenance can also be seen as investments in embodied capital. Thus, the present-future reproductive trade-off can be understood in terms of optimal investments in own embodied capital vs. reproduction, and the quantity-quality tradeoff can be understood in terms of investments in the embodied capital of offspring vs. their number.

The Brain as Embodied Capital

The brain is a special form of embodied capital. Neural tissue is involved in monitoring the organism's internal and external environment and organizing physiological and behavioral adjustments to those stimuli (Jerison 1976). Portions (particularly the cerebral cortex) are also involved in transforming present experiences into future performance. Cortical expansion among higher primates, along with enhanced learning abilities, reflects increased investment in transforming present experience into future performance (Armstrong and Falk 1982; Fleagle 1999).

The action of natural selection on neural tissue involved in learning and memory should depend on costs and benefits realized over the organism's lifetime. Three kinds of costs are likely to be of particular importance. First, there are the initial energetic costs of growing the brain. Among mammals, those costs are largely born by the mother. Second, there are the energetic costs of maintaining neural tissue. Among infant humans, about 65 % of all resting energetic expenditure supports maintenance and growth of the brain (Holliday 1978). Third, certain brain capacities may actually decrease performance early in life. Specifically, the ability to learn and increased behavioral flexibility may entail reductions in "pre-programmed" behavioral routines. The incompetence with which human infants and children perform many motor tasks is an example.

Some allocations to investments in brain tissue may provide immediate benefits (e.g., perceptual abilities, motor coordination). Other benefits of brain tissue are only realized as the organism ages. The acquisition of knowledge and skills has benefits that, at least in part, depend on their impact on future productivity. Figure 1 illustrates two alternative cases, using as an example the difficulty and learning-intensiveness of the organism's foraging niche. In the easy feeding niche, where there is little to learn and little information to process, net productivity (excess energy above and beyond maintenance costs of brain and body) reaches its asymptote early in life. There is a relatively small impact of the brain on productivity late in life (because there is little to learn), but there are higher costs of the brain early in life. Unless the life span is exceptionally long, natural selection will favor the smaller brain.

In the difficult food niche, the large-brain creature is slightly worse off than the small-brain one early in life (because the brain is costly and learning is taking place), but much better off later in life. The effect of natural selection will depend upon the probabilities of reaching the older ages. If those probabilities are sufficiently low, the small brain will be favored; if they are sufficiently high, the large brain will be favored. Thus, selection on learning-based neural capital

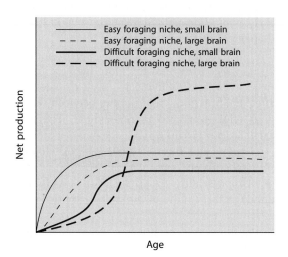

Fig. 1. Age-specific effects of brains on net production: easy and difficult foraging niches

depends not only on its immediate costs and benefits but also upon mortality schedules that affect the expected gains in the future.

Selection on Mortality Schedules

In standard LHT models, mortality is generally divided into two types: 1) extrinsic mortality (i.e., mortality, such as predation or winter, that is imposed by the environment and is outside the control of the organisms) and 2) intrinsic mortality (hazards of mortality over which the organism can exert some control over the short run or that are subject to selection over the longer periods). In most models of growth and development, mortality is treated as extrinsic (Charnov 1993; Kozlowski and Wiegert 1986) and therefore as a causal agent, not subject to selection. Models of aging and senescence (Promislow 1991; Shanley and Kirkwood 2000) typically focus on aging-related increases in intrinsic mortality. Extrinsic mortality, in turn, is thought to affect selection on rates of aging, with higher mortality rates favoring faster aging.

This distinction between types of mortality is problematic. Organisms can exert control over virtually all causes of mortality in the short- or long-run. Susceptibility to predation can be affected by vigilance, choice of foraging zones, travel patterns and anatomical adaptations, such as shells, cryptic coloration and muscles facilitating flight. Each of those behavioral and anatomical adaptations has energetic costs (lost time foraging, investments in building and maintaining tissue) that reduce energy available for growth and reproduction. Similar observations can be made regarding disease and temperature. The extrinsic mortality concept has been convenient because it has provided a causal agent for examining other life history traits, such as age of first reproduction and rates of aging. However, this has prevented the examination of how mortality rates themselves evolve by natural selection.

Since all mortality is, to some extent, intrinsic or "endogenous", a more useful approach is to examine the functional relationship between mortality and effort allocated to reducing it (see Fig. 2). Exogenous variation can be thought of in terms of varying "assault" types and varying "assault" rates of mortality hazards. For example, warm, humid climates favor the evolution of disease organisms and therefore increase the assault rate and diversity of diseases in organisms living in those climates. Such exogenous variation would affect the functional relationship between actual mortality hazards and endogenous effort allocated to reducing it. The outcome mortality rate is neither extrinsic nor intrinsic.

Kaplan and Robson (2001 a, b) developed formal models to analyze the simultaneous effects of natural selection on both investments in capital and in reducing mortality. As a first step, it is useful to think of capital generally (interpreted as the bundle of functional abilities embodied in the soma). Organisms generally receive some energy from their parents (e.g., in the form of energy stored in eggs) to produce an initial stock of capita. Net energy acquired from the environment at each age grows as a function of the capital stock, with

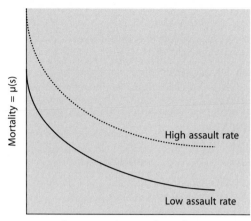

Fig. 2. Mortality rate as a function of investments

diminishing returns to capital (as illustrated in Fig. 3). This energy can be used in three ways that are endogenous and subject to selection. It can be reinvested in increasing the capital stock (e.g., growth of the body or brain). Some energy may also be allocated to reducing mortality (for example in the form of increased immune function, as illustrated above in Fig. 2). The probability of reaching any age will be a function of mortality rates at each earlier age. Finally, energy can also be used for reproduction, which is the net excess energy available after allocations to capital investments and mortality reduction. An optimal life history program would optimize allocations to capital investments, mortality reduction, and reproduction at each age so as to maximize total energy allocations to reproduction over the life course. This, of course, depends both on reproductive allocations and on survival.

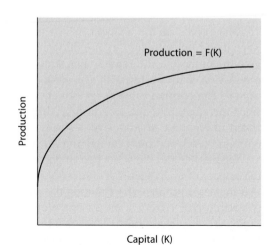

Fig. 3. Production as a function of the capital stock. At each point in time, an individual has an embodied capital stock, K, that produces a stream of energy output, F (K). The stock grows during development

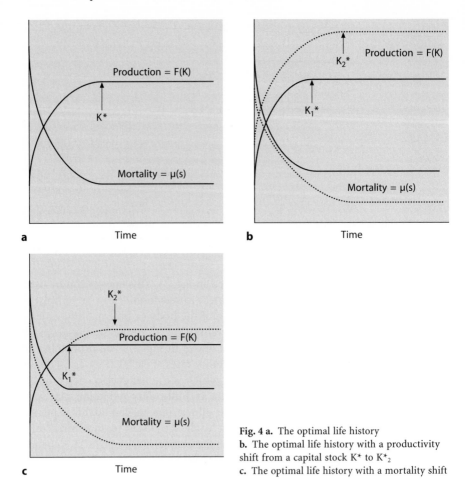

Fig. 4 a. The optimal life history
b. The optimal life history with a productivity shift from a capital stock K* to K*₂
c. The optimal life history with a mortality shift

The results of the analysis, which are presented and proven formally in Kaplan and Robson (2001 a), are illustrated in Figures 4 a–c. During the capital investment period, the value of life, which is equal to total expected future net production, is increasing with age, since productivity is growing with increased capital. The optimal value of investment in mortality reduction also increases, since the effect of a decrease in mortality increases as capital increases (illustrated in Fig. 4 a). At some age, a steady state is reached when capital is at its optimum level, and both capital and mortality rates remain constant.

Figures 4 b and 4 c show two important comparative results. In Figure 4 b, the impact of a change in productivity is shown. Some environmental change that increases productivity (holding the marginal value of capital constant) has two reinforcing effects: it increases the optimal level of both capital investment (and hence the length of the investment period) and efforts to reduce mortality. Figure 4 c shows the impact of a reduction in mortality rates, again with two effects. It both increases the optimal capital stock (because it increases the expected length of life and hence the time over which it will yield returns) and produces a reinforcing increase in effort at reducing mortality, since the impact of a decrease in mortality is greater as mortality rates decrease.

Finally, the model shows that a shift in productivity from younger to older ages (for example, an increased reliance on learning that lowers juvenile energy production but increases adult production) increases the value of living to older ages and therefore the optimal effort at reducing mortality. This has the effect of increasing expected life span. Our theory is that brain size and longevity co-evolve for the following reasons. Ecological conditions favoring large brains also select for greater endogenous investments in staying alive. As the stock of knowledge and functional abilities embodied in the brain grow with age, so too does the value of the capital investment. This favors greater investments in health and mortality avoidance. In addition, holding the value of the brain constant, ecological conditions that lower mortality select for increased investment in brain capital for similar reasons; an increased probability of reaching older ages increases the value of investments whose rewards are realized at older ages. The next section applies this logic to the brain and life span evolution in the primate order.

Brain and Life Span Evolution among Primates

The Theoretical and Empirical Model

Relative to other mammalian orders, the primate order can be characterized as slow-growing, slow-reproducing, long-lived and large-brained. The radiation of the order over time has involved a series of four directional grade shifts towards slowed life histories and increased encephalization (i.e., brain size relative to body size). Even the more "primitive" prosimian primates are relatively long-lived and delayed in reaching reproductive maturity compared to mammals of similar body size, which suggests the same of early primate ancestors. Austad and Fischer (1991, 1992) relate this evolutionary trend in the primates to the safety provided by the arboreal habitat and compare primates to birds and bats, which are also slow-developing and long-lived for their body sizes. Thus, the first major grade shift that separated the primate order from other mammalian orders was a change to a lowered mortality rate and the subsequent evolution of slower senescence rates, leading to longer life spans and slightly larger brains.

The second major grade shift occurred with the evolution of the anthropoids (the lineage containing monkeys, apes and humans), beginning about 35 mya. Its major defining characteristic is the reorganization of the sensory system, one dominated by binocular, color vision and associated with hand-eye coordination as opposed to olfaction and hearing. These sensory changes co-occurred with an increased emphasis on plant foods (especially hard seeds and fruits), as opposed to insects (Benefit 2000; Fleagle 1999). The grade shift is also seen in brain size and life history. Regressions of log brain size on log body size (Barton 1999), as well as log maximum life span on body size (Allman et al. 1993), show significant differences in intercept between strepsirhine (including most prosimians) and haplorhine (including all anthropoids and a few prosimians) primates. Relative to prosimians, anthropoids also have lower metabolic rates and longer gestation times (Martin 1996).

The evolution of monkey and ape dietary adaptations in the Miocene and Pliocene appears to be based on an early adaptation for both groups to feed on hard seeds and green fruits (Benefit 2000). In the Late Miocene/Early Pliocene, cercopithecoids, which had been semi-terrestrial, cursorial, hard seed and green fruit eaters much like modern vervet monkeys, evolved new digestive adaptations allowing the colobines to digest mature leaves. Cercopithecoids also began to more directly compete with apes in both terrestrial and arboreal habitats. Miocene apes were highly diverse and found in many habitats but were essentially agile arboreal quadrupeds. By the Late Miocene apes had fully developed their characteristic shoulder girdle morphology, allowing suspension below branches that gave special access to ripe fruits for larger bodied animals. This dietary shift to dependence on ripe fruits, based on the morphological adaptation of arm suspension, moved apes into a new grade with an emphasis on feeding higher in the food pyramid on very nutritious food packets high in energy but spatially and temporally dispersed in an arboreal habitat. This new grade reduced direct competition with monkeys, ceded open terrestrial habitat to them, and greatly reduced the number and diversity of ape species. At the same time it put a premium on acquired knowledge about the location of ripe fruits and for skills for more complex extractive foraging of embedded and protected, high energy and fatty foods such as nuts, insects and hard-shelled fruits.

This third major grade shift marked the evolution of the hominoid lineage (leading to apes and humans). This grade shift entailed further encephalization, as revealed by a yet greater intercept of log brain size regressed on log body size and superior performance on most tasks reflecting higher intelligence (Byrne 1995 b; Byrne 1997 b; Parker and McKinney 1999). The divergence of the hominid line, and particularly the evolution of genus *Homo*, defines the fourth major grade shift. The brain size and life span of modern humans are very extreme values among mammals, and even primates. Although the record is incomplete, it appears that brain enlargement and life history shifts co-occurred. Early *Home ergaster* shows both significant brain expansion and a lengthened developmental period (Smith 1993), but much less to than modern humans. Neanderthals display both brain sizes and dental development that are in the same range as modern humans. Modern humans have a brain size about three times that of female gorillas of similar weight, and about double the maximum life span.

The proposal here is that both shifts in mortality risks and in the benefits of information storage and processing due to changes in feeding niche underlie these directional changes in the primate lineage through time. However, in addition to these large-scale shifts, a great deal of adaptive variation exists

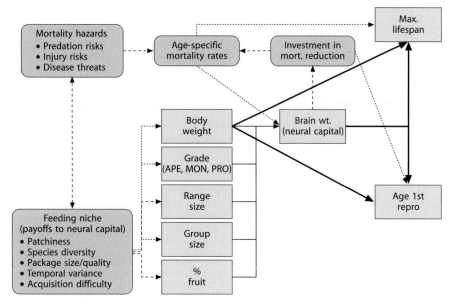

Fig. 5. A theoretical and empirical path model of primate brain evolution. MON, monkey; PRO, prosimian

among primates. Species of all four grades continue to co-exist, often sympatrically (especially monkeys, apes and humans). Moreover, not all evolutionary change has been in the direction of larger brains and longer lives. For example smaller-brained monkeys appear to have replaced apes in some niches at the end of the Miocene (Benefit 2000; Fleagle 1999). If changes in mortality risks and the learning intensiveness of the feeding niche explain the grade shifts, the same factors might also explain variation within grades.

Figure 5 illustrates the theory and the empirical model that it generates, given the available data. On the left, the two rounded boxes represent exogenous ecological variables.[1] Some features of the feeding niche that are likely to affect the payoffs to information acquisition and processing (and hence, brain size) are listed in the lower box. Resource patchiness tends to be associated with larger home ranges and potentially greater demands on spatial memory. The number of different species consumed potentially adds to demands for spatial memory, learned motor patterns, processing of resource characteristics, and temporal associations (Jerison 1973). Large, nutrient-dense, packages (such as big, ripe fruits) tend to be patchily distributed in space and often with very short windows of availability (Clutton-Brock and Harvey 1980; Milton 1981, 1993). Year-to-year abundance and location of high-quality packages also

---

[1] Although feeding niche is subject to selection, the suites of foods eaten are treated as givens in order to model how selection molds life history traits, brain size and other features of phenotype in response to niche conditions.

appear to vary. Hence, diets with a greater relative importance of large, high-quality packages are probably associated with increased brain size through several routes: by increasing the number of species exploited, by increasing the size of the home range, and by increasing the importance of predicting the timing and location of availability. In addition, some high quality foods, such as hard-shelled fruits, nuts, insects, and honey, must be extracted from protective casings and their exploitation often requires learned strategies and tools.

Features of the environmental/behavioral niche of the organism that are likely to affect mortality rates and the payoffs of investments in mortality reduction are listed in the upper, left box. Life in or near trees probably increases injury risk but decreases predation risk to overall lower mortality risks. Lowered risk of mortality due to predation is expected to increase investment in combating disease and, hence, decrease disease risks as well (though these have received little attention in primate studies to date). Lower mortality rates increase the probability of reaching older ages and therefore affect the payoffs to larger brains, holding feeding niche constant.

The co-evolution of brain size and mortality patterns is shown in the path diagram (dashed arrows depict effects of unmeasured conceptual or latent variables). Both features of the feeding niche and mortality risks affect optimal brain size. Brain size is expected to have both direct and indirect effects on life span and age of first reproduction. Larger brains may confer direct survival advantages through increased physiological efficiency and through learned predator avoidance (Allman et al. 1993; Armstrong 1982; Hakeem et al. 1996; Jerison 1973; Rose and Mueller 1998). In addition, since larger brains are associated with greater relative productivity at older ages, brain size is expect to be associated with investment in mortality reduction. Similarly, the energetic costs of the brain reduce energy available for growth, and learning-based feeding niches may lower productivity during the juvenile period. This would produce slower growth rates and a later age of first reproduction, holding body size constant. The greater allocations to mortality reduction (e.g., increased immune function, reduced foraging time) would also slow the growth rates.

The rectangular boxes depict measured variables for which comparative data are available, and the solid arrows depict associations that can be tested empirically. The thinner lines represent the first stage in the model, predicting brain weight. Measures of feeding niche are captured by grade (ape, monkey vs. prosimian), range size, and percentage of fruit in the diet. We also include body and group size in this first stage. In addition to directly affecting brain size, body size is likely to be associated with dietary niche. For example, larger home ranges probably favor larger bodies, because of their greater locomotor efficiency. Larger home ranges may also be associated with larger groups, because holding resource abundance constant, a patchy environment will tend to produce both larger home ranges and a larger number of individuals feeding at each resource patch (Wrangham 1979). Because the social intelligence hypothesis has figured so prominently in the literature (Barton and Dunbar 1997; Byrne 1995 b; Dunbar 1998), the path between group size and brain size is also

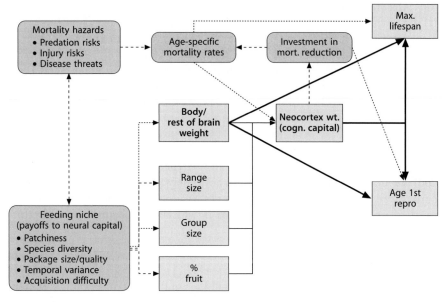

Fig. 6. A theoretical and empirical path model of neocortex evolution

included. In addition, if social intelligence takes time to acquire and its benefits are weighted towards older ages (as may well be the case), embodied capital theory does predict that selection on social intelligence will co-evolve with longevity and mortality rates. For example, social intelligence might allow alpha males to retain their high status to older ages and it might confer greater benefits to females when they have many descendants (in the case of ranked matrilines). Such effects would also be consistent with the model. The second stage, shown with bold arrows, examines the effects of brain size and body size on age of first reproduction and maximum recorded life span, respectively.

A second model will also be tested (see Fig. 6). The logic of the embodied capital model suggests that the brain functions that are most involved in transforming present experience into future performance should have the greatest impact on the payoffs to living longer and allocating effort to mortality reduction. In addition, it has been argued that the association of brain size with life span in primates, after controlling for body size, is spurious and due to greater measurement error in body size than in brain size [Dunbar 1998; Economos 1980, although Allman et al. (1993) have shown that brain size is a better predictor of life span than the size of other organs]. To address these issues, the size of the neocortex will be disaggregated from the rest of the brain. The neocortex should better reflect the learning intensiveness of the feeding niche and social system than the rest of the brain. In the second model, neocortex weight replaces brain weight, and the weight of the rest of the brain replaces body weight, as an instrument (since measurement error for neocortex and rest of brain weight, respectively, should be similar).

The Primate Sample

Data are available on the total adult brain weights (in grams) for 124 species, compiled from secondary sources (Barton 1999; Harvey et al. 1987). From this sample, there are 95 species for which data are available on mean adult body weight (in grams), group size, age at first breeding for females (in months), maximum life span (in years), maximum home range (in hectares), and percent frugivory. Much of the data came from secondary sources (Barton 1996, 1999; Dunbar 1992; Harvey et al. 1987; Ross 1992). These data differ, however, from previous analyses in a heavier reliance on primary field data for female age at first breeding, maximum home range, and percent frugivory (see Kaplan et al. 2001 for details). They may thus more accurately represent the selection pressures faced by wild individuals, which are assumed to be living in conditions much more representative of the context in which these features co-evolved.

Results

A two-stage least squares regression analysis was performed to test the models. For the model in Figure 5, the first stage was conducted hierarchically. First, the natural logarithm of brain weight was regressed on the natural logarithms of body weight, range size, and group size, and on percent age of fruit in the diet. Then to capture other aspects of niche differentiation, grade (ape and monkey, compared to a prosimian baseline) was added as a fixed effect to determine if it significantly improved the model. The results are presented in Table 1. In the simple model without grade, body weight, range size and percent age of fruit in the diet are each positively related to brain weight, accounting for 94 % of the variance. Group size was not significant. Grade significantly improved the model fit ($p < .0001$), with the model now accounting for 97 % of the variance. In this model, percent age of fruit is no longer significant, but group size is. The predicted values of log brain size from this full model are then used in the second stage of the analysis.[2]

Part B of Table 1 shows the results of the second stage, in which the natural logarithms of female age at first reproduction and maximum reported life span, respectively, are regressed on the logs of predicted brain weight and body weight. In both cases, brain weight explains most of the variance and the effect of body weight is now negative. When brain weight is not in the model, the association between body weight and both life span and age of first reproduction is, of course, strongly positive. It may be that, after controlling for brain weight, larger bodied species eat lower quality diets (Aiello and Wheeler 1995; Milton 1981, 1987, 1988, 1993; Milton and Demment 1988), and this is associated with a relatively shorter life span and earlier age at first reproduction.

---

[2] Since brain size is endogenous, the problem of simultaneity can be addressed by using predicted brain size in this second regression. Similar results are obtained, however, when measured values are used instead of predicted values.

Table 1. Two-stage model of brain size and life history

A. Stage I, brain weight

Parameter	B	Std. Error	t	Sig.	B	Std. Error	t	Sig.
		$R^2 = 0.94$, N = 95				$R^2 = 0.97$, N = 97		
Intercept	−1.74	0.16	−11.22	0.0000	−1.74	0.16	−11.22	0.0000
Body weight	0.68	0.03	23.01	0.0000	0.59	0.02	24.83	0.0000
Range size	0.05	0.03	1.95	0.0550	0.05	0.02	2.54	0.0130
Group size	0.07	0.04	1.64	0.1040	0.07	0.04	2.02	0.0468
Percentage fruit	0.00	0.00	2.65	0.0100	0.00	0.00	1.46	0.1484
Ape	–	–	–	–	0.87	0.10	8.73	0.0000
Monkey	–	–	–	–	0.45	0.07	6.42	0.0000
Prosimian	–	–	–	–	0.00	–	–	–

B. Stage II

Parameter	B	Std. Error	t	Sig.	B	Std. Error	t	Sig.
		Maximum life span, $R^2 = 0.52$, N = 80				Age of first reproduction, $R^2 = 0.74$, N = 79		
Intercept	3.14	0.34	9.32	0.0000	2.78	0.37	7.58	0.0000
Body weight	−0.24	0.10	−2.36	0.0208	−0.21	0.11	−1.99	0.0503
Brain weight	0.53	0.13	4.12	0.0001	0.71	0.14	5.19	0.0000

The results of decomposing brain weight into the neocortex and the rest of the brain (Fig. 6) are shown in Tables 2 and 3. Using the same set of regressors as in the full model of brain size, the natural logarithms of the weights of rest of the brain and of the neocortex (shown on the left and right sides of Table 2, respectively) are each treated as dependent variables. Body weight and grade are the only variable that significantly affects the weight of non-neocortical brain tissue, and the effect of grade is rather small. With respect to neocortex

Table 2. Neocortex and rest of brain weight

Parameter	B	Std. Error	t	Sig.	B	Std. Error	t	Sig.
		Rest of brain weight (Brain weight–Neocortex weight) $R^2 = 0.94$, N = 32				Neocortex weight, $R^2 = 0.98$, N = 32		
Intercept	−2.03	0.30	−6.66	0.0000	−2.46	0.25	−9.68	0.0000
Body weight	0.55	0.05	10.42	0.0000	0.57	0.04	13.02	0.0000
Range size	0.08	0.04	1.79	0.0860	0.12	0.04	3.41	0.0020
Group size	−0.05	0.07	−0.68	0.5010	0.02	0.06	0.28	0.7800
Percentage fruit	0.00	0.00	0.42	0.6810	0.00	0.00	0.77	0.4470
Ape	0.51	0.23	2.25	0.0330	0.89	0.19	4.64	0.0000
Monkey	0.27	0.16	1.73	0.0950	0.71	0.13	5.51	0.0000
Prosimian	0.00	–	–	–	0.00	–	–	–

Table 3. Two-stage model of neocortex size and life history

Stage I

Parameter	B	Std. Error	t	Sig.
		Neocortex size, $R^2 = 0.996$, N = 32		
Intercept	−0.26	0.05	−5.03	0.0000
Rest of brain weight	1.10	0.03	31.83	0.0000
Range size	0.01	0.02	0.76	0.4556
Group size	0.06	0.03	2.35	0.0270
Percentage fruit	0.00	0.00	0.88	0.3871
Ape	0.52	0.09	5.99	0.0000
Monkey	0.47	0.06	8.29	0.0000
Prosimian	0.00	–	–	–

Stage II

Parameter	B	Std. Error	t	Sig.
		Maximum life span, $R^2 = 0.70$, N = 32		
Intercept	2.66	0.11	25.21	0.0000
Rest of brain weight	−0.20	0.24	−0.83	0.4122
Neocortex weight	0.38	0.19	2.05	0.0506
		Age of first reproduction, $R^2 = 0.79$, N = 32		
Intercept	2.49	0.14	17.42	0.0000
Rest of brain weight	−0.30	0.31	−0.99	0.3304
Neocortex weight	0.64	0.24	2.69	0.0119

weight, however, both range size and grade have large effects. Thus, consistent with the above logic, feeding niche has a larger effect on neocortex weight than on the rest of the brain, which appears to be more a function of body weight.

In Table 3, the weight of the rest of the brain is used as an instrument for body weight in stage 1 of the model. This model shows that neocortical weight increases more than proportionally with the rest of the brain (b = 1.1), and that both grade and group size have large significant effects. In the second stage, predicted neocortical weight is positively associated with both age at first reproduction and maximum life span, whereas the rest of the brain is not significantly associated with the life history variables. This finding is also consistent with the model. These results should be treated with some caution, however, because the two measures of brain weight are highly collinear.

The Evolution of *Homo*: Chimpanzees and Modern Humans Compared

The same principles may explain the very long lives and the very large brains characteristic of the genus *Homo* and particularly of modern *Homo sapiens*. *Homo* has existed for about 2 million years. Figure 7 shows that human ances-

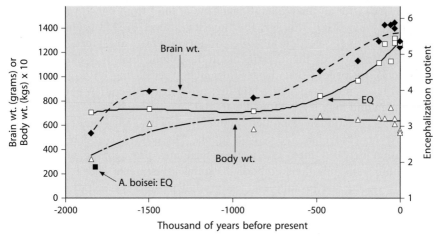

Fig. 7. Hominid brain size and body weight. EQ, encephalization quotient

tors experienced a dramatic increase in brain size but a much less marked increase in body size, especially during the second half of this period. Using Martin's (Martin 1981) measure of "Encephalization Quotient *(EQ)*" (i.e., brain weight corrected allometrically for body weight, with $EQ = \dfrac{(brain\ wt)}{11.22^* \ (body\ wt.)^{.76}}$; one is the average value for a mammal), the large increases in brain size relative to body size are shown with the bold line. Australopithecus, the presumed evolutionary ancestor of *Homo*, coexisted with early *Homo*. *A. boisei*, in particular, had an *EQ* of just over two, which compares to about 3.5 for early *Homo*. Life spans of extinct species are not directly observable, of course, but indirect evidence suggests the life span of australopithecines was much less than that of modern humans and comparable to that of chimpanzees (Smith 1991), with early species in the genus *Homo* having life spans (Smith 1993) that are intermediate between chimpanzees and modern humans.

Hominids have subsisted on hunting and gathering, perhaps supplemented by scavenging, for all but the last 10,000 years of our evolutionary history. Our proposal (see Kaplan + Robson 2002; Kaplan 1997; Kaplan et al. 2000) is the hunting and gathering lifestyle is responsible for the evolution of these extreme values with respect to brain size and longevity. Our proposal is that large brains and long lives are co-evolved responses to an equally extreme commitment to learning-intensive foraging strategies and a dietary shift towards high-quality, nutrient-dense, and difficult-to-acquire food resources. The following logic underlies our proposal. First, high levels of knowledge, skill, coordination and strength are required to exploit the suite of high-quality, difficult-to-acquire resources humans consume. The attainment of those abilities requires time and a significant commitment to development. This extended learning phase during which productivity is low is compensated for by higher productivity during the adult period, with an intergenerational flow of food from old to young. Since productivity increases with age, the time investment in skill acquisition and knowledge leads to selection for lowered mortality rates and greater longevity, because the returns on the investments in development occur at older ages.

Second, we believe that the feeding niche specializing on large, valuable food packages, and particularly hunting, promotes cooperation between men and women and high levels of male parental investment, because it favors sex-specific specialization in embodied capital investments and generates a complementarity between male and female inputs. The economic and reproductive cooperation between men and women facilitates provisioning of juveniles, which both bankrolls their embodied capital investments and acts to lower mortality during the juvenile and early adult periods. Cooperation between males and females also allows women to allocate more time to childcare and increases nutritional status, increasing both survival and reproductive rates. Finally, large packages also appear to promote inter-familial food sharing. Food sharing assists recovery in times of illness and reduces risk of food shortfalls due to both the vagaries of foraging luck and to variance in family size due to stochastic mortality and fertility. These buffers against mortality also favor a longer juvenile period and higher investment in other mechanisms to increase life span.

Thus, the proposal is that the long human life span co-evolved with the lengthening of the juvenile period, increased brain capacities for information processing and storage, and intergenerational resource flows – all as a result of an important dietary shift. Humans are specialists in that they only consume the highest quality plant and animal resources in their local ecology and rely on creative, skill-intensive techniques to exploit them. Yet, the capacity to develop new techniques for extractive foraging and hunting allows them to exploit a wide variety of different foods and to colonize all of the Earth's terrestrial and coastal ecosystems.

The best available evidence for evaluating this theory is to compare wild living chimpanzees, human's closest living relatives, with contemporary hunter-gatherers who still subsist on foraging for subsistence and who have little or no access to Western medicine. Both chimpanzees and contemporary foragers have been affected by current global trends, such as deforestation, population movements, and other effects of modern economies. They cannot be treated as replicas of the evolutionary past. Nevertheless, the differences in the diets, survival rates, and age profiles of productivity between chimpanzees and contemporary hunter-gatherers are striking and consistent with the theory.

Diet, Survival and Age Profiles of Productivity among chimpanzees and contemporary hunter-gatherers

Diet

There are ten foraging societies[3] and five chimpanzee communities for which caloric production or time spent feeding were monitored systematically (Kaplan et al. 2000). Modern foragers all differ considerably in diet from chimpanzees. Measured in calories, the major component of forager diets is vertebrate meat, which ranges from about 30 % to around 80 % of the diet in the sampled societies, with most diets consisting of more than 50 % vertebrate meat (equally weighted mean = 60 %), whereas chimpanzees obtain about 2 % of their food energy from hunted foods.

The next most important food category in the forager sample is extracted resources, such as roots, nuts, seeds, most invertebrate products, and difficult-to-extract plant parts, such as palm fiber or growing shoots. They may be defined as non-mobile resources that are embedded in a protective context such as underground, in hard shells or bearing toxins that must be removed before they can be consumed. In the ten-forager sample, extracted foods accounted for about 32 % of the diet, as opposed to 3 % among chimpanzees.

In contrast to hunted and extracted resources, which are difficult to acquire, collected resources form the bulk of the chimpanzee diet. Collected resources, such as fruits, leaves, flowers, and other easily accessible plant parts, are simply gathered and consumed. They account for 95 % of the chimpanzee diet, on average, and only 8 % of the forager diet.

The data suggest that humans specialize in rare but nutrient-dense resource packages or patches (meat, roots, nuts) whereas chimpanzees specialize in ripe fruit and low-nutrient-density plant parts. These differences in nutrient density of foods ingested are also reflected in human and chimpanzee gut morphology and food passage time, with chimpanzees specialized for rapid processing of large quantities and low nutrient, bulky, fibrous meals (Milton 1999).

The Age Profile of Acquisition for Collected, Extracted, and Hunted Resources

In most environments, fruits are the easiest resources that people acquire. Daily production data among Ache foragers show that both males and females reach their peak daily fruit production by their mid to late teens. Some fruits that are simply picked from the ground are collected by two- to three-year-olds at 30 % of the adult maximum rate. Ache children acquire five times as many calories

---

[3] The hunter-gatherer data come from studies on populations during periods when they were almost completely dependent on wild foods, with little modern technology (and no firearms), no significant outside interference in interpersonal violence or fertility rates, and no significant access to modern medicine (see Kaplan et al. 2000 for details).

per day during the fruit season as during other seasons of the year (Kaplan 1997). Similarly, among the Hadza, teen girls acquired 1650 calories per day during the wet season, when fruits were available, and only 610 calories per day during the dry season, when fruits were not. If we weight the wet and dry season data equally, Hadza teen girls acquire 53 % of their calories from fruits, compared to 37 % and 19 % for reproductive-aged and post-reproductive women, respectively (Hawkes et al. 1989).

In contrast to fruits, the acquisition rate of extracted resources often increases through early adulthood as foragers acquire necessary skills. Data on Hiwi women show that root acquisition rates do not asymptote until about age 35–45 (Kaplan et al. 2000) and the rate of 10-year-old girls is only 15 % of the adult maximum. Hadza women appear to obtain maximum root digging rates by early adulthood (Hawkes et al. 1989). Hiwi honey extraction rates by males peak at about age 25. Again the extraction rate of 10-year-olds is less than 10 % of the adult maximum. Experiments done with Ache women and girls clearly show that young adult girls are not capable of extracting palm products at the rate obtained by older Ache women (Kaplan et al. 2000). Ache women do not reach peak return rates until their early 20s.! Kung (Ju/'hoansi) children crack mongongo nuts at a much slower rate than adults (Blurton Jones et al. 1994), and Bock (1995) has shown that nut-cracking rates among the neighboring Hambukushu do not peak until about age 35. Finally, chimpanzee juveniles also focus on more easily acquired resources than adult chimpanzees. Difficult-to-extract activities such as termite and ant fishing or nut cracking are practiced less by chimpanzee juveniles than by adults (Boesch and Boesch 1999; Hiraiwa-Hasegawa 1990; Silk 1978).

Human hunting differs qualitatively from hunting by other animals and is the most skill-intensive foraging activity. Unlike most animals that either sit and wait to ambush prey or use stealth and pursuit techniques, human hunters use a wealth of information to make context-specific decisions, both during the search phase of hunting and then after prey are encountered. Specifically, information on ecology, seasonality, current weather, expected animal behavior and fresh animal signs is all integrated to form multivariate mental models of encounter probabilities that guide the search and are continually updated as conditions change (Leibenberg 1990). Various alternative courses of action are constantly compared and referenced to spatial and temporal mental maps of resource availability (ibid). This information is collected, memorized and processed over much larger spatial areas than chimpanzees ever cover. For example, interviews with Ache men show that fully adult men (aged 35+) had hunted in an area of nearly 12,000 km^2 of tropical forest in their lifetimes. Almost all foragers surveyed use more than 200 km^2 in a single year, and many cover more than 1000 km^2 in a year (Kelly 1995; Table 4.1). Male chimpanzees, on the other hand, cover only about 10 km^2 in a lifetime (Wrangham and Smuts 1980; Wrangham 1975).

In addition, humans employ a wide variety of techniques to capture and kill prey, using astounding creativity (Kaplan et al. 2000). Those kill techniques are tailored to many different prey under a wide variety of conditions. For example, from 1980 to 1996 our sample of weighed prey among the Ache includes a minimum of 78 different mammal species, at least 21 species of reptiles and amphibians, probably over 150 species of birds (more than we have been able to identify) and over 14 species of fish. Finally, human hunters tend to select prey that is in prime condition from the perspective of human nutritional needs rather than prey made vulnerable by youth, old age or disease as do so many carnivorous animals (Alvard 1995; Stiner 1991).

The skill-intensive nature of human hunting and the long learning process involved are demonstrated dramatically by data on hunting return rates by age. Hunting return rates among the Hiwi do not peak until age 30–35, with the acquisition rates of 10-year-old and 20-year-old boys reaching only 16 % and 50 % of the adult maximum, respectively. The hourly return rate for Ache men peaks in the mid 30s. The return rate of 10-year-old boys is about 1 % of the adult maximum, and the return rate of 20-year-old juvenile males is still only 25 % of the adult maximum. Marlowe (unpublished data) obtained similar results for the Hadza. Also, boys switch from easier tasks, such as fruit collection, shallow tuber extraction and baobab processing, to honey extraction and hunting in their mid to late teens among the Hadza, Ache and Hiwi (Blurton Jones et al. 1989, 1997; Kaplan et al. 2000). Even among chimpanzees, hunting is strictly an adult or subadult activity (Boesch and Boesch 1999; Stanford 1998; Teleki 1973).

Survival and Net Food Production

Figure 8 (Kaplan et al. 2000) shows the probabilities of survival and net production (i.e., food acquired minus food consumed) by age. The chimpanzee net production curve shows three distinct phases. The first phase, to about age five, is the period of complete to partial dependence upon mother's milk and of negative net production. The second phase is independent juvenile growth, lasting until adulthood, during which net production is zero. The third phase is reproductive, during which females, but not males, produce a surplus of calories that they allocate to nursing.

Humans, in contrast, produce less than they consume for about 20 years. Net production becomes increasing by negative until about age 14 and then begins to climb. Net production in adult humans is much higher than in chimpanzees and peaks at a much older age, reflecting the payoff of long dependency. More precisely, human peak net production is about 1750 calories per day, reached at about age 45. Among chimpanzee females, peak net production is only about 250 calories per day and, since fertility decreases with age, net productivity probably decreases throughout adulthood.

The survival curves, using the scale on the right-hand y-axis, reveal why the human age profile of productivity requires a long adult life span. Only about 30 % of chimpanzees ever born reach 20, the age when humans produce as

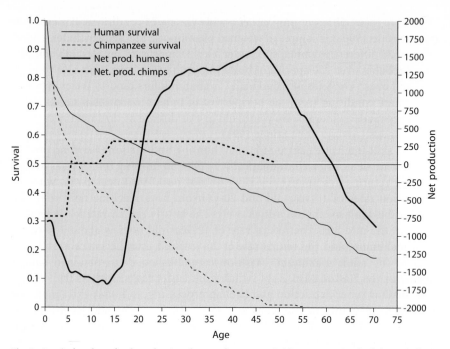

Fig. 8. Survival and net food production: human foragers and chimpanzees. On the left vertical axis is the probability of survival and on the right is net production in calories per day. The data on chimpanzee survival are derived from averaging age-specific mortality rates from all five study sites where systematic data on births and deaths are recorded (Hill et al. 2001); data on chimpanzee food consumption and production are from Gombe (Goodall 1986). Human survival rates are averaged from Ache (Hill and Hurtado 1996), Hiwi (Kaplan et al. 2000), and Hadza (Blurton Jones et al. 2002). Net production data are from the same groups (details on all sources and estimation procedures for both human and chimpanzee production and consumption data are in Kaplan et al. 2000

much as they consume. Less than 5% of chimpanzees reach 45, when human net production peaks, but more than 15% of hunter-gatherers survive to age 70. By age 15, chimpanzees have consumed 43% and produced 40% of their expected lifetime calories, respectively; in contrast, humans have consumed 22% and produced only 4% of their expected lifetime calories!

The relationship between survival rates and age profiles of production is made even clearer in Figure 9. The thin solid line plots net production by age for foragers (as in Fig. 8). The bold line shows expected net production for foragers, which is net production at each age multiplied by the probability of being alive at each age. The area of the "deficit" period, prior to age 20, is about the same size as the surplus after age 20. The dashed line shows the hypothetical "contrary to fact" expected net production profile of a human forager with a chimpanzee survival function. The area of the deficit is now much larger than the area of the surplus, since very few individuals survive to the highly productive ages. This shows that the human production profile would not be viable with chimpanzee survival rates, because expected lifetime net production would be negative.

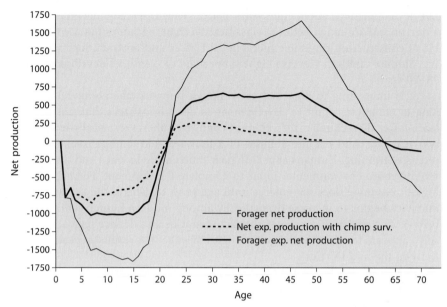

Fig. 9. Expected net production

Development and Cognitive Function Among Monkeys, Apes and Humans

Although human intelligence has long been recognized as our most distinctive specialization as a species, it is now becoming increasing clear that our larger brains and greater intellectual capacities depend upon the elongation or stretching out of development at every stage. The production of cortical neurons in mammals is limited to early fetal development and, compared to monkeys and apes, human embryos spend an additional 25 days in this phase (Deacon 1997; Parker and McKinney 1999). The greater original proliferation of neurons in early fetal development has cascading effects in greatly extending other phases of brain development, ultimately resulting in a larger, more complex and effective brain. For example, in monkeys, such as macaques, myelination of the brain begins prenatally and is largely complete in three month, but in humans continues to at least 12 years of age (Gibson 1986). Dendritic development is similarly extended to age 20 or greater in humans.

The timing of cognitive development is extended in chimpanzees relative to monkeys and in humans relative to apes (Parker and McKinney 1999). In terms of Piagetian stages, frequently used by comparative cognitive psychologists, macaque monkeys traverse only two sub-periods of cognitive development regarding physical phenomena by about six months of age and peak in their logical abilities by about three years of age; however, they fail to be able to represent objects symbolically, to classify objects hierarchically or to recognize themselves in a mirror. Chimpanzees traverse three to four subperiods of cognitive development by about eight years of age.[4] They can recognize themselves in a mirror and are much better at classification than macaques but are not capable of constructing reversible hierarchical classes and abstract, logical reasoning. Human children traverse eight subperiods of cognitive development over 18–20 years.

It is interesting to note that even though humans take about 2.5 times as long to complete cognitive development as do chimpanzees, humans actually learn faster than chimpanzees. In most cognitive spheres, especially language, a two-year-old child has the abilities of a four-year-old chimpanzee, even with intensive training. Humans appear to have much more to learn and their brains require more environmental input to complete development. Formal abstract logical reasoning does not emerge until age 16 to 18. This is the age when productivity begins to increase dramatically among modern hunter-gatherers (see below). The ability to construct abstract scenarios and deduce logical relationships appears to allow for the growth in knowledge that results in peak productivity in the mid thirties.

Elongated development in humans is also associated with slowed aging of the brain. Macaques exhibit physiological signs of cognitive impairment, as evidenced by the appearance of Alzheimer-like neuropathology (senile plaques, neurocytoskeletal abnormalities) and cerebral atrophy by age 22–25, and chimpanzees by age 30, in contrast to humans for whom such changes are rare until age 60 (< 1%) and only common (> 30%) by age 80s (Finch 2002).

Mechanisms Underlying Brain-Longevity Co-Evolution

There are several possible pathways by which, at the species level, brain size and function might co-evolve with life span and the process of aging. One possibility is simply through the additive phenotypic effects of genes contributing to the selective environment of other genes. For example, the phenotypic effects of genes affecting brain development and function increase foraging returns for high-quality, nutrient-dense foods during adulthood. The ensuing diet and age profile of production then constitute the selective environment for genes affecting dietary physiology (e.g., the size of the large intestine) and rates of aging (e.g., accumulation of plaque and free radicals). At the same time, those phenotypic effects of those latter genes affect the selective environment for genes affecting brain tissue and brain development. This could result in a "ratcheting" process, in which both sets of genes change over time, resulting in nonrandom associations of brains and longevity at the species level.

Another possibility is that such associations could be due to pleitropy (i.e., single genes influencing more than one trait) and/or linkage disequilibrium (sets of genes jointly assorting during meiosis). Research into brain aging and

---

[4] The fourth subperiod, such as conservation of quantities of liquids under container transformations, seem to require tutelage and symbolic training.

longevity suggests that some genes may have such pleiotropic effects. The apolipo-protein (apoE) allele system is a good example since this seems to affect neurite growth and the aging of both the brain and the cardiovascular system. (The discussion here is based on Finch and Sapolsky 1999, which gives the original sources.) Brain aging, as in the symptoms of Alzheimer's disease, is common in long-lived mammals. These signs of brain aging are delayed in humans relative to apes and in apes relative to monkeys. In humans, apoE has at least three variants (apoE ε2, ε3 and ε4) whereas all nonhuman primates that have been studied have the same variant, most similar to human apoE ε4. Interestingly, this variant is a risk factor for both Alzheimer's disease and coronary artery disease, suggesting that the apoE ε2 and ε3 variants may have evolved to slow down both brain and cardiovascular aging. These other variants also promote neurite growth in cultured neurons, suggesting they also stimulate greater brain development and complexity.

Pleitropic effects of this nature could evolve by a similar ratcheting process. The sensitivity of one tissue type (e.g., neurons) to a gene product could affect selection on sensitivity of other tissue types (e.g., vascular tissue) to that same gene product, and vice versa. To the extent that associations between brains and longevity are due to pleitropic effects, this would generate correlations at the individual level as well as at the species level. Given the growing body of data suggesting that such individual-level associations exist among humans, pleitropy deserves careful consideration.

Another possible pathway underlying associations at the individual level, especially among humans, is through adaptive behavioral flexibility. Human life histories, including the life span, show evidence of systematic variation in response to environmental variation. Those effects appear to be the result of the interaction between changes in environmental conditions and human physiology and behavior. Perhaps the most dramatic example of that interaction is the pattern of changes accompanying modernization, the secular trend. Increased nutrition and decreased disease loads have systematic effects on human developmental physiology. Physical growth rates increase and maturation begins earlier, resulting in greater stature, higher body weight and earlier age of menarche in girls (Eveleth 1986; Lancaster 1986; Worthman 1999). This response is very likely the result of selection on adaptive flexibility in growth and maturation due to environmental variation in food supply and disease assault rates experienced during human evolutionary history.

In contrast to this increase in physical developmental rate, aging may be slowed in response to better nutrition and decreased disease loads. Although it is possible that humans would also show slowed aging in response to radical reductions in caloric intake (Shanley and Kirkwood 2000), it is also possible that under the more common range of variation, rates of aging are slowed and life spans are longer when nutrition is better and disease loads are lower (Fogel and Costa 1997), and this too is adaptive. The changing mortality rates among older people accompanying modernization and the fact that many chronic diseases occurred at earlier ages in the 19th century U.S. than today (Costa 2000) are consistent with such a possibility.

One countervailing force may also be the product of adaptive flexibility to past environmental variation. Increased risk of heart disease, diabetes and cancer due to overweight and lack of exercise may also be the result of evolved responses. Given the common activity regimes in our past and the variability in food supply, human appetites and nutritional biochemistry may be designed to store fat and increase blood lipid levels when food is abundant. Those adaptations may be acting to shorten the life span in the context of modern activity regimes and food access.

In addition to these physiological adaptations, there are also behavioral responses to modernization. The models outlined in Figures 2–4 are equally applicable to short-term behavioral variation as they are to long-term life history adaptations. Two dramatic effects of modernization are increased economic payoffs to educational capital and decreased mortality due to improvements in public health. Those models predict reinforcing endogenous behavioral responses to such changes. Increased payoffs to education should promote both increased investment in educational capital and in staying alive. Improvements in public health should also promote reinforcing increases in capital investment and staying alive. The fact that income grows more with age with increasing education suggests that there will be similar differentiation across educational groups. Thus, individuals with high levels of education and intelligence may expect their economic status to grow as they age, and therefore engage in behavior that increases their likelihood of reaching older ages; conversely, those whose future prospects seem poor or not likely to improve with age might be less inclined to invest in health. Similarly, variation in exposure to risks of mortality (associate with violence, AIDS, or other hazards) should affect willingness to invest in education and future earnings.

Discussions and Conclusions

The analyses in this paper have applied embodied capital theory to understanding primate radiations in brain size and longevity and the evolution of the human life course. Embodied capital theory organizes the relationships of ecology, brain size and longevity among primates, which existing debates about primate brain size evolution have failed to do. Most studies of brain evolution have ignored longevity and focused either on the benefits or on the costs of brains, but not both. The liveliest current debate concerns whether the benefit of a large brain is to solve ecological or social problems (Allman et al. 1993; Barton and Dunbar 1997; Byrne and Whiten 1988; Clutton-Brock and Harvey 1980; Dunbar 1998; Milton 1993). On the cost side, another debate concerns, for example, whether larger brains require smaller guts or lower metabolic rates (Aiello and Wheeler 1995; Barton 1999; Foley and Lee 1991; Martin 1996).

Studies examining the relationship between the brain and longevity fail to model simultaneous selection. One focus has been on whether the relationship between brain size and longevity is real or a statistical artifact (Allman et al.

1993; Barton 1999; Economos 1980; Foley and Lee 1991; Martin 1996). Another has been on the metabolic costs of growing large brains (Foley and Lee 1991; Martin 1996) and its indirect relationship to life span through body size. Others have focused either on the direct impacts of the brain on life span or on the benefits of a longer life span. For example, Sacher (1975) offers two proposals: 1) brains directly increase life span by ensuring more precise homeostasis of bodily functions; and 2) brains delay maturation and lower the reproductive rate, therefore requiring an extension of the life span. Other hypotheses are: 1) larger brains are beneficial to longer-lived animals because they are likelier to experience food shortages when knowledge of the habitat would facilitate survival (Allman et al. 1993); 2) larger brains decrease ecological vulnerability to environmental risks and select for increased longevity (Rose and Mueller 1998); and 3) larger brains help maintain tissue differentiation and slow the process of entropy leading to senescence (Hofman 1983).

The embodied capital theory shows how features of ecology, including both mortality risks and information processing demands, interact in determining optimal allocations to the brain and survival. It also suggests an alternative interpretation of primate social intelligence. Co-evolutionary selection on brains and longevity due to the complexity and the navigational demands of the primate diet may have produced pre-adaptations for the evolution of social intelligence. Given that primates live long lives with enduring social relationship and given that many species of primates eat foods whose distribution generates within-group competition, there would be selection for the application of existing enhancements in memory and information processing abilities to the management of social interaction. Many animals live in social groups, but primates are notable in terms of the complexity of their social arrangements. Perhaps social pressures alone are not sufficient to select for markedly increased brain size, but they might select for the extension of existing abilities to social problems. This may be why apes display remarkable social intelligence, even though group size is not particularly large (Byrne 1995 a, 1997 a). Orangutans, for example, are mostly solitary, but it takes about seven years for a young orangutan to become independent of its mother (presumably because of the learning-intensive nature of the diet). If this view is correct, it also suggests that the assumption of extreme domain specificity in intelligence may be unwarranted.

There is growing interest in the evolution of human life histories, especially longevity. One model, recently proposed by Hawkes and colleagues (Hawkes et al. 1998), often referred to as the "Grandmother Hypothesis", proposes that humans have a long life span because of the assistance that older, post-reproductive women contribute to descendant kin through the provisioning of difficult-to-acquire plant foods. Women, therefore, are selected to invest in maintaining their bodies longer than chimpanzee females. This model offers no explanation why men live so long. In contrast to this female-centered view, Marlowe (2000) proposes that reproduction by males late in life selects for the lengthening of the human life course, with effects on females being incidental.

The embodied capital theory explains why both men and women live long lives. Both men and women exploit high quality, difficult-to-acquire foods (females extracting plant foods and males hunting animal foods), sacrificing early productivity for later productivity, with a life history characterized by an extended juvenile period where growth is slow and much is learned, and a high investment in mortality reduction to reap the rewards of those investments.

The human adaptation is broad and flexible, in one sense, and very narrow and specialized, in another sense. It is broad in the sense that, as hunter-gatherers, humans have existed successfully in virtually all of the world's major habitats. This has entailed eating a very wide variety of foods, both plant and animal, and a great deal of flexibility in the contributions of different age- and sex-classes of individuals. The human adaptation is narrow and specialized in that it is based on extremely high investments in brain tissue and learning. In every environment, human foragers consume the largest, highest quality, and most difficult-to-acquire foods, using techniques that often take years to learn. It is this legacy that modern humans bring to the complex economies existing today, where education-based embodied capital determines income and the economy is a complex web of specialization and cooperation between spouses, families and larger social units. We are only beginning to explore the implications of this legacy for understanding modern behavior.

References

Aiello L, Wheeler P (1995) The expensive-tissue hypothesis: The brain and the digestive system in human and primate evolution. Curr Anthropol 36: 199–221

Allman J, McLaughlin T, Hakeem A (1993) Brain weight and life-span in primate species. Proc Nat Acad Sci pp. 118–122

Alvard M (1995) Intraspecific prey choice by Amazonian hunters. Curr Anthropol 36: 789–818

Armstrong E (1982) A look at relative brain size in mammals. Neurosci Lett 34: 101–104

Armstrong E, Falk D (eds) (1982) Primate brain evolution. New York: Plenum Press

Austad SN, Fischer KE (1991) Mammalian aging, metabolism, and ecology: evidence from the bats and marsupials. J Gerontol 46: 47–51

Austad SN, Fischer KE (1992) Primate longevity: Its place in the mammalian scheme. Am J Primatol 28: 251–261

Barton RA (1996) Neocortex size and behavioral ecology in primates. Proc Roy Acad (Biol Sci) 263: 173–177

Barton RA (1999) The evolutionary ecology of the primate brain. In: Lee PC (ed) Comparative primate socioecology. Cambridge: Cambridge University Press, pp. 167–203

Barton RA, Dunbar RIM (1997) Evolution of the social brain. In: Whiten A, Byrne RW (eds) Machiavellian Intelligence II. Cambridge: Cambridge University Press, pp. 240–263

Benefit BR (2000) Old World monkey origins and diversification: An evolutionary study of diet and dentition. In: Whitehead P, Jolly CJ (eds) Old World monkeys. Cambridge: Cambridge University Press, pp. 133–179

Blurton Jones N, Hawkes K, O'Connell J (1989) Modeling and measuring the costs of children in two foraging societies. In: Standen V, Foley RA (eds) Comparative socioecology of humans and other mammals. London: Basil Blackwell, pp. 367–390

Blurton Jones NG, Hawkes K, Draper P (1994) Foraging returns of !Kung adults and children: Why didn't !Kung children forage? J Anthropol Res 50: 217–248

Blurton Jones NG, Hawkes K, O'Connell J (1997) Why do Hadza children forage? In: Segal NL, Weisfeld GE, Weisfield CC (eds) Uniting psychology and biology: integrative perspectives on human development. New York: Am Psychol Assoc pp. 297–331

Blurton Jones NB, Hawkes K, O'Connell J (2002) The antiquity of post-reproductive life: Are there modern impacts on hunter-gatherer post-reproductive lifespans? Human Biol 14: 184–205

Bock JA (1995) The determinants of variation in children's activities in a Southern African Community. Ph. D. Dissertation, University of New Mexico, Albuquerque

Boesch C, Boesch H (1999) The chimpanzees of the Tai forest: behavioral ecology and evolution. Oxford: Oxford University Press

Byrne RW (1995 a) The smart gorilla's recipe book. Nat Hist Oct: 12–15

Byrne RW (1995 b) The thinking ape: the evolutionary origins of intelligence. Oxford: Oxford University Press

Byrne RW (1997 a) Machiavellian intelligence. In: Whiten A, Byrne RW (eds) Machiavellian intelligence II: extensions and evaluations. Cambridge: Cambridge University Press, pp. 1–23

Byrne RW (1997 b) The technical intelligence hypothesis: an additional evolutionary stimulus to intelligence? In: Whiten A, Byrne RW (eds): Machiavellian intelligence II: extensions and evaluations. Cambridge: Cambridge University Press, pp. 289–311

Byrne RW, Whiten A (eds) (1988) Machiavellian intelligence. Oxford: Clarendon Press

Charnov EL (1993) Life history invariants: some explanations of symmetry in evolutionary ecology. Oxford: Oxford University Press

Clutton-Brock TH, Harvey PH (1980) Primates, brains and ecology. J Zool London 109: 309–323

Cole LC (1954) The population consequences of life history phenomena. Quart Rev Biol 29: 103–137

Costa DL (2000) Understanding the twentieth century decline in chronic conditions among older men. Demography 37: 53–72

Deacon TW (1997) The symbolic species. New York: W. W. Norton & Co

Dunbar RIM (1992) Neocortex size as a constraint on group size in primates. J Human Evol 20: 469–493

Dunbar RIM (1998) The social brain hypothesis. Evol Anthropol 6: 178–190

Economos AC (1980) Brain-life span conjecture: A re-evaluation of the evidence. Gerontology 26: 82–89

Eveleth PB (1986) Timing of menarche: Secular trend and population differences. In: Lancaster JB, Hamburg BA (eds) School-age pregnancy and parenthood. Hawthorne, NT: Aldine de Gruyter, pp. 39–53

Finch CE (2002) Evolution and the plasticity of aging in the reproductive schedules in long-lived animals: The importance of genetic variation in neuroendocrine mechanisms. In: Pfaff D, Arnold A, Etgen A, Fahrback S, Rubin R (eds) Hormones, brain and behavior. San Diego: Academic Press

Finch CE, Sapolsky RM (1999) The evolution of Alzheimer disease, the reproductive schedule and the apoE isoforms. Neurobiol Aging 20: 407–428

Fleagle JG (1999) Primate adaptation and evolution. New York: Academic Press

Fogel RW, Costa DL (1997) A theory of technophysio evolution, with some implications for forecasting population, health care costs and pension costs. Demography 34: 49–66

Foley RA, Lee PC (1991) Ecology and energetics of encephalization in human evolution. Phil Trans Roy Soc London B 334: 63–72

Gadgil M, Bossert WH (1970) Life historical consequences of natural selection. Am Naturalist 104: 1–24

Gibson KR (1986) Cognition, brain size and the extraction of embedded food resources. In: Else JG, Lee PC (eds) Primate ontogeny, cognition, and social behavior. Cambridge: Cambridge University Press, pp. 93–105

Goodall J (1986) The chimpanzees of the Gombe: patterns of behavior. Cambridge: Cambridge University Press

Hakeem A, Sandoval GR, Jones M, Allman J (1996) Brain and life span in primates. In: Abeles RP, Catz M, Salthouse TT (eds) Handbook of the psychology of aging. San Diego: Academic Press, pp. 78–104

Harvey PH, Martin RD, Clutton-Brock TH (1987) Life histories in comparative perspective. In: Smuts BB, Cheney DL, Seyfarth RM, Wrangham RW, Struthsaker TT (eds) Primate societies. Chicago: University of Chicago

Hawkes K, O'Connell JF, Blurton Jones N (1989) Hardworking Hadza grandmothers. In: Standen V, Foley RA (eds) Comparative socioecology of humans and other mammals. London: Basil Blackwell, pp. 341–366

Hawkes K, O'Connell JF, Blurton Jones NG, Alvarez H, Charnov EL (1998) Grandmothering, menopause, and the evolution of human life histories. Proc Nat Acad Sci USA 95: 1336–1339

Hill K, Hurtado AM (1996) Ache life history: the ecology and demography of a foraging people. Hawthorne, NY: Aldine

Hill K, Boesch C, Goodall J, Pusey A, Williams J, Wrangham R (2001) Mortality rates among wild chimpanzees. J Human Evol 39: 1–14

Hiraiwa-Hasegawa M (1990) The role of food sharing between mother and infant in the ontogeny of feeding behavior. In: Nishida T (ed) The chimpanzees of the Mahale Mountains: sexual and life history strategies. Tokyo: Tokyo University Press, pp. 267–276

Hofman MA (1983) Energy metabolism, brain size and longevity in mammals. Quart Rev Biol 58: 495–512

Holliday MA (1978) Body composition and energy needs during growth. In: Falker F, Tanner JM (eds) Human growth. New York: Plenum Press, pp. 117–139

Jerison H (1973) Evolution of the brain and intelligence. New York: Academic Press

Jerison HJ (1976) Paleoneurology and the evolution of mind. Sci Am 234: 90–101

Kaplan HS (1997) The evolution of the human life course. In: Wachter K, Finch C (eds) Between Zeus and salmon: the biodemography of aging. Washington, D.C.: Natl Acad Sci, pp. 175–211

Kaplan H, Robson A (2001 a) The coevolution of intelligence and life expectancy in hunter-gatherer economies. London, Ontario: Department of Economics, University of Western Ontario

Kaplan H, Robson A (2001 b) The co-evolution of intelligence and lifespan and the emergence of humans. Albuquerque, NM: Department of Anthropology, University of New Mexico

Kaplan H, Robson A. in press. "The evolution of life expectancy and intelligence in hunter-gatherer economies." American Economic Review.

Kaplan H.S, A. Robson. 2002. "The emergence of humans: The coevolution of intelligence and longevity with intergenerational transfers." Proceedings of the National Academy of Sciences 99: 10221–10226.

Kaplan H, Hill K, Hurtado A.M, Lancaster J.B, Robson A. in press. "Embodied capital and the evolutionary economics of the human lifespan." Population and Development Review, Supplement.

Kaplan HS, Hill K, Lancaster JB, Hurtado AM (2000) A theory of human life history evolution: Diet, intelligence, and longevity. Evol Anthropol 9: 156–185

Kaplan HS, Gangestad S, Mueller TC, Lancaster JB (2001) The evolution of primate brains and life histories: A new model and empirical analysis. Albuquerque, NM: University of New Mexico

Kelly RL (1995) The foraging spectrum: Diversity in hunter-gatherer lifeways. Washington, D.C.: Smithsonian Institution Press

Kozlowski J, Wiegert RG (1986) Optimal allocation to growth and reproduction. Theoret Pop 29: 16–37

Lack D (1954) The natural regulation of animal numbers. Oxford: Oxford University Press

Lancaster JB (1986) Human adolescence and reproduction: An evolutionary perspective. In: Lancaster JB, Hamburg BA (eds) School-age pregnancy and parenthood. Hawthorne, NY: Aldine de Gruyter, pp. 17–39

Leibenberg L (1990) The art of tracking: the origin of science. Cape Town: David Phillip

Lloyd DG (1987) Selection of offspring size at independence and other size-versus-number strategies. Am Naturalist 129: 800–817

Marlowe F (2000) The patriarch hypothesis: An alternative explanation of menopause. Human Nat 11, pp. 27–42

Martin RD (1981) Relative brain size and basal metabolic rate in terrestrial vertebrates. Nature 293: 57–60

Martin RD (1996) Scaling of the mammalian brain: The maternal energy hypothesis. News Physiol Sci 11: 149–156

Milton K (1981) Distribution patterns of tropical plant foods as an evolutionary stimulus to primate mental development. Am Anthropol 83: 534–548

Milton K (1987) Primate diet and gut morphology: implications for human evolution. In: Harris M, Ross EB (eds) Food and evolution: toward a theory of human food habits. Philadelphia: Temple University Press, pp. 93–116

Milton K (1988) Foraging behaviour and the evolution of primate intelligence. In: Byrne RW, Whiten A (eds) Machiavellian intelligence. Oxford: Clarendon Press, pp. 285–305

Milton K (1993) Diet and primate evolution. Sci Am 269: 70–77

Milton K (1999) A hypothesis to explain the role of meat-eating in human evolution. Evol Anthropol 8: 11–21

Milton K, Demment M (1988) Digestive and passage kinetics of chimpanzees fed high and low fiber diets and comparison with human data. J Nutrit 118: 107

Parker ST, McKinney ML (1999) Origins of intelligence: the evolution of cognitive development in monkeys, apes and humans. Baltimore: Johns Hopkins Press

Partridge L, Harvey P (1985) Costs of reproduction. Nature 316: 20–21

Promislow DEL (1991) Senescence in natural populations of mammals: A comparative study. Evolution 45: 1869–1887

Rose MR, Mueller LD (1998) Evolution of the human lifespan: past, future and present. Am J Human Biol 10: 409–420

Ross C (1992) Basal metabolic rate, body weight and diet in primates: An evaluation of the evidence. Folia Primatol 58: 7–23

Sacher GA (1975) Maturation and longevity in relation to cranial capacity in hominid evolution. In: Tuttle R (ed) Primate functional morphology and evolution. The Hague: Mouton, pp. 417–441

Shanley DP, Kirkwood TBL (2000) Calorie restriction and aging: a life-history analysis. Evolution 54: 740–750

Silk JB (1978) Patterns of food-sharing among mother and infant chimpanzees at Gombe National Park, Tanzania. Folia Primatol 29: 129–141

Smith BH (1991) Dental development and the evolution of life history in Hominidae. Am J Physical Anthropol 86: 157–174

Smith BH (1993) The physiological age of KNM-WT 15 000. In: Walker A, Leakey R (eds) The Nariokotome Homo erectus skeleton. Cambridge: Harvard University Press, pp. 196–220

Smith CC, Fretwell SD (1974) The optimal balance between size and number of offspring. Am Naturalist 108: 499–506

Stanford CB (1998) Chimpanzee and Red Colobus: the ecology of predator and prey. Cambridge, MA: Harvard University Press

Stiner M (1991) An interspecific perspective on the emergence of the modern human predatory niche. In: Stiner M (ed) Human predators and prey mortality. Boulder: Westview Press, pp. 149–185

Teleki G (1973) The predatory behavior of wild chimpanzees. Lewisburg, PA: Bucknell University Press

Worthman CM (1999) Evolutionary perspectives on the onset of puberty. In: Trevathan WR, Smith EO, McKenna JJ (eds) Evolutionary medicine. Oxford: Oxford University Press, pp. 135–163

Wrangham RW (1979) On the evolution of ape social systems. Soc Sci Info 18: 335–368

Wrangham RW, Smuts B (1980) Sex differences in behavioral ecology of chimpanzees in Gombe National Park, Tanzania. J Reprod Fertil (Suppl) 28: 13–31

Wrangham W (1975) The behavioral ecology of chimpanzees in Gombe National Park, Tanzania. Ph.D. dissertation, Cambridge University, Cambridge

How did longevity promote brain expansion during primate evolution?

S. I. Rapoport

Summary

Evidence indicates that cognitive ability, brain size and life span co-evolved during primate evolution. It is not difficult to conceive how prolongation of the initial phases of the life span – gestation, infancy and adolescence and young
adulthood – contributed to this co-evolution. Prolonged gestation would have
provided larger brains at birth, whereas prolonged infancy, adolescence and
young adulthood would have extended brain neuroplasticity to allow experience and learning to modify brain structure in individuals (genotypes) faced
with new cognitive and social stresses, making them more competitive and
reproductively successful. Natural selection in primates also involved genetically related kinships. Through cooperation within kinships, older genotypes
who were most cognitively and socially competitive because of their larger
brains could contribute to the success of their kin, indirectly extending their
own genes in the general population. In some cases, a new longer-lived, more
cognitively-capable, larger-brained primate species appeared.

Introduction

> "Alone a youth runs fast; with an elderly person, slowly; but together they
> go far."
>
> Luo Saying, Kenya

Studies of longevity have largely asked why some species live longer than other
species, or why some individuals within a species live longer than other individuals. One cause for these differences is genetic, as longevity has been shown in
some species to be regulated by specific genes, some of which are involved in
energy metabolism (Gems and Partridge 2001; Martin 1996; Puca et al. 2001;
Van Voorhies and Ward 1999). Differences in expression of longevity genes
probably account for differences in life span among moth species, in which of
older individuals can contribute to survival (Blest 1963). Another cause for life
span differences likely is differences in metabolism. Among mammalian species, a lower basal metabolic rate is associated with a longer life expectancy
(Hofman 1983 b, 1989; Rasmussen and Izard 1988). This finding has been

Finch et al. (Eds.)
Brain and Longevity
© Springer-Verlag Berlin Heidelberg 2003

ascribed to the fact that oxidative metabolism produces reactive oxygen species (ROS), which can shorten life span by damaging protein and DNA or increasing the mutation rate (Beckman and Ames 1998; Campisi 2000; Harman 1992; Sohal and Weindruch 1996; Wallace 1992). Thus, reduced caloric intake has been shown to prolong life span of individuals within some species by reducing energy metabolism and the ROS load. Superoxide dismutase/catalase mimetics, which inactivate ROS, can do so as well (Melov et al. 2000).

In *Origin of Species*, Charles Darwin identified three necessary conditions for promoting speciation: population variation of individual traits that are heritable, environmental stress, and natural selection of individuals most capable of competing in the stressful environment (Darwin 1859). Natural selection allows the most competitively successful individuals, or "genotypes," to best reproduce so as to extend their genes in the population gene pool, in some cases leading to a new species (Medawar and Medawar 1983; Rapoport 1999). In this context, longevity would be a neutral fitness factor[1] because older genotypes would be less competitive and less likely to reproduce (Fischer 1958; Kimura 1983; Michod 1999). Thus, they would "escape the force of natural selection" (Martin 2001; Medawar 1955).

On the other hand, in this paper I suggest that longevity was a positive fitness factor for co-evolution of brain, cognition and life span in primates, because a unit of natural selection in primates was the kinship of genetically related individuals as well as the individual. Thus, older, less successfully reproductive primates could nevertheless have their genes extend in the species population by enhancing the competitiveness and reproductive success of their kin. Depending on their brain size and function, they could accomplish this by increasing the information storage, judgment, and cognitive and social strategies of the kinship, and by contributing to social cohesiveness and flexibility, training and child rearing, adjudication of conflict and reduced social tension.

Correlation Between Life Span Phases, Brain Size and Cognitive-Social Abilities During Primate Evolution

Brain anatomy. As illustrated in Table 1, mean brain weight relative to body weight increased during primate evolution, particularly in the last five million years of hominid speciation. As the primate brain expanded, two internal "systems" of association regions were elaborated. The first system includes association neocortex and connected areas of hippocampus, amygdaloid complex, cin-

---

[1] Fitness can be represented as the rate of increase of an index i (e.g., gene or gene-related phenotypic characteristic) in successive generations. In this context, selection may be said to occur when the frequency of the property q_i after selection, f_i^c, is greater than the frequency f_i before selection. Thus, a positive fitness factor can be identified as a ratio of f_i^c to f_i, exceeding 1, a neutral factor as causing a ratio of 1, and a negative factor as decreasing the ratio to below 1.

Table 1. Endocranial volume and body weight in primates[a]

Family Species	Endocranial volume (Mean (range), cm^3)	Body weight (kg)	Time of appearance (millions of years)
Lemur	26	2.2	
Cebus	67	3.1	26
Macaque	88	7.8	8
Hylobates	98	5.7	19
Gorilla	470	105	8
Pan troglodytes	383 (282–500)	47	7.5–6.5
Pan paniscus	343 (275–381)	35	3.1–2.5
Hominids			
Australopithecus afarensis	401	24	> 4–2.5
Australopithecus africanus	442 (428–486)	36	3.2–2.2
Homo habilis	644 (590–687)	42	2.5–1.5
Homo erectus javanicus	926 (813–1059)	49	1.8–0.6
Homo erectus pekinensis	1043 (915–1225)	53	0.7–0.5
Homo sapiens (neanderthalis)	1487 (1200–1750)	83	> 0.22
Modern Homo sapiens	1365 (1156–1775)	9	0.2

[a] Values are from fossil record except for modern Homo sapiens and Pan. Remaining values are from living species. Data from: Campbell 1988; Cann et al. 1987; Deacon 1992; Dunbar 1992; Hofman 1983 a; Jones et al. 1992; Martin 1990

gulate cortex and entorhinal cortex. The second system includes other parts of association neocortex, as well as thalamus, basal ganglia and subcortical catecholaminergic nuclei (Rapoport 1990).

Intelligence. There is no accepted way to compare intelligence test scores among different primate species (Rumbaugh and Pate 1984; Tomasello and Call 1997). However, it is generally recognized that the great apes (chimpanzees, gorillas and orangutans) have an intellectual capacity between modern *Homo sapiens* and simians. The great apes, like modern humans, are capable of self-recognition and can easily learn to use complex tools. *Pan paniscus* (Bonobos) and perhaps other great apes can learn to manipulate visual lexigrams according to syntactic rules, and like humans their brains demonstrate hemispheric asymmetry with expansion of a region corresponding to Broca's language area in the left hemisphere. These higher-order abilities, as well as spoken language in humans, are best learned during "critical periods" of development, when certain brain regions are most sensitive to permanent modulation (Ameli 1980; Beck 1975; Cantalupo and Hopkins 2001; Gallup 1977; Matsuzawa 1994; Newport 1990; Povinelli and Eddy 1996; Rumbaugh and Pate 1984; Rumbaugh et al. 1996; Savage-Rumbaugh et al. 1993; Whiten et al. 1999).

Longevity. As illustrated by Figure 1, life span increased in relation to the appearance of new species of primates (Dehay et al. 1993; Gould 1977; Lovejoy 1981, Pagel and Harvey 1988). Increased life span was accompanied by a roughly proportional prolongation of each of its phases: gestation, infancy, adolescence, adulthood and post-reproductive senescence (in humans). This

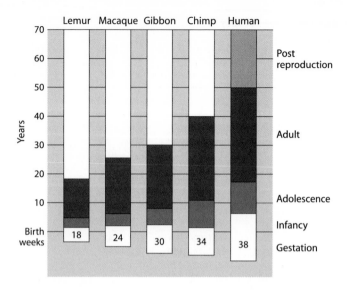

Fig. 1. *Prolongation of life span phases in primates in relation to order of speciation* (from Lovejoy 1981)

proportionality likely reflects the influence throughout life of longevity-regulating genes or of the level of basal metabolism (see above).

How Did Prolongation of the Initial Phases of the Life Span Promote Brain Growth During Primate Evolution?

Based on the principles of natural selection of individuals (Darwin 1871; Darwin 1859), it is not difficult to imagine how extension of each life phase except for late adulthood promoted co-evolution of brain and cognition in primates:

Gestation. Prolongation of gestation would have produced larger brains at birth by allowing more time for pre-natal mitotic division and production of neurons and glia (Gould 1977; Rapoport 1999). For example, a single extra round of mitotic division at the stage of formation of proliferative units at the ventricular surface of the neutral tube (before stage E40 in the human fetus) would double the number of available cortical neurons formed from these units (Rakic 1988). Supporting a role for prolonged gestation on brain evolution is evidence that neocortical brain size at birth and gestation length are correlated in living mammalian species (Pagel and Harvey 1988).

Infancy and adolescence. Prolongation of infancy and adolescence would have allowed the brain to remain highly neuroplastic for longer periods, and thus more easily modified by experience and learning in individuals faced with new cognitive or social stresses. Intense neuroplasticity during infancy and adolescence in primates is accompanied by marked synaptic proliferation and pruning and expression of growth factors (Constantine-Paton 1990; Feinberg 1983; Gould et al. 2000; Huttenlocher 1990; Huttenlocher 1979; Huttenlocher and Dabholkar 1997; Knipper et al. 1997; Rakic et al. 1986; Rapoport 1999). Neuroplasticity also is present in the adult primate brain, albeit to a lesser extent than during development (Beck et al. 2000; Benowitz et al. 1989; Cabelli et al. 1995; Gould et al. 2000; Hatanpää et al. 1999; Holden 1997; Neve et al. 1988).

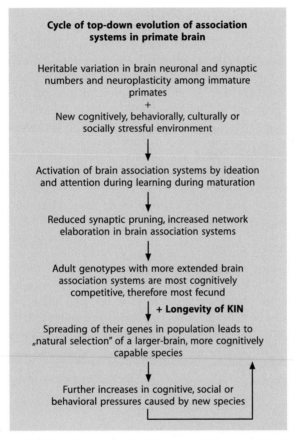

Cycle of top-down evolution of association systems in primate brain

Heritable variation in brain neuronal and synaptic numbers and neuroplasticity among immature primates
+
New cognitively, behaviorally, culturally or socially stressful environment

↓

Activation of brain association systems by ideation and attention during learning during maturation

↓

Reduced synaptic pruning, increased network elaboration in brain association systems

↓

Adult genotypes with more extended brain association systems are most cognitively competitive, therefore most fecund

↓ **+ Longevity of KIN**

Spreading of their genes in population leads to „natural selection" of a larger-brain, more cognitively capable species

↓

Further increases in cognitive, social or behavioral pressures caused by new species

Fig. 2. *Feedback model for "top-down" evolution of brain association systems in primates.* The model assumes that higher order thought and attentional processes, free of sensory input, can directly activate widespread brain regions in immature primates. Activation will lead to optimization of the brain "association" networks that are most capable of enhancing the cognitive and social ability of the genotype. Selection takes place when a genetically heterogeneous population is faced with new cognitive, social, cultural or behavioral stresses. The genes of the successful adults spread within the population, leading in some cases to a new cognitively and socially more competent, larger-brained species. This process is recursive (upward arrows at bottom of figure provide feedback mechanism), as a newer larger-brained species will create additional cognitive or behavioral stresses (Whiten et al. 1999; Wilson 1985). The figure also illustrates, as a, of +, highlighted positive modulation by longevity of large-brained cognitively competent but nonfecund individuals of the reproductive rates of kin with whom they share critical genes (see text) (adapted from Rapoport 1999)

Figure 2 illustrates a proposed "top-down" scenario for the natural selection of larger-brained primates. The scenario is based on the neuroplastic capacity of the developing brain to be permanently modified by experience and learning (Rapoport 1999). In this scenario, a population is suddenly faced with new cognitive and social stresses. Those younger individuals (genotypes) who are best able to adapt to these stresses, because of their larger, more neuroplastic brain, will be most competitive and reproductively successful as adults. Their genes thereby will extend in the species population, giving rise in some cases to a new, more cognitively able, larger-brained species. This new species in turn may engender more intense cognitive or social pressures, leading to further natural selection of even more brain-competent individuals. Such a "positive feedback" scenario appears to have accelerated during the last five million years of hominid speciation (Table 1). It is consistent with evidence that neocortical volume correlates with group size (representing social pressure) among living primate genera (Fig. 3) (Dunbar 1992 b).

Two recently solidified concepts are consistent with the "top-down" process shown in Figure 2 (Rapoport 1999). 1) Functional activation of the immature neuroplastic brain can expand and stabilize neuronal networks and synaptic connections that underlie cognition and behavior (Changeux 1983). 2) Independently of sensory input, higher order cognitive processes such as ideation and attention can activate wide areas of primate brain. Thus thinking of a boat may activate the same visual areas as seeing a picture of a boat. This internally initiated ("top-down") activation has been experimentally demonstrated in nonhuman primates and humans by means of *in vivo* imaging and direct brain recording (Fig. 4) (Corbetta et al. 1991; Hinke et al. 1993; Kosslyn et al. 1995, 1999; Mellet et al. 1996; Roland 1982). Putting these two concepts together, it is not difficult to accept that brain networks underlying higher order cognition and behavior can be activated, thus elaborated and stabilized, by ideation and attention and other thought processes, so as to maximize the individual's ability to adapt to cognitive and social stresses in his environment.

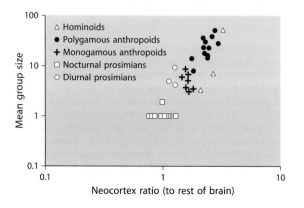

Fig. 3. *Mean group size for individual genera plotted against neocortex ratio (volume neocortex to rest of brain)* (from Dunbar 1992 b)

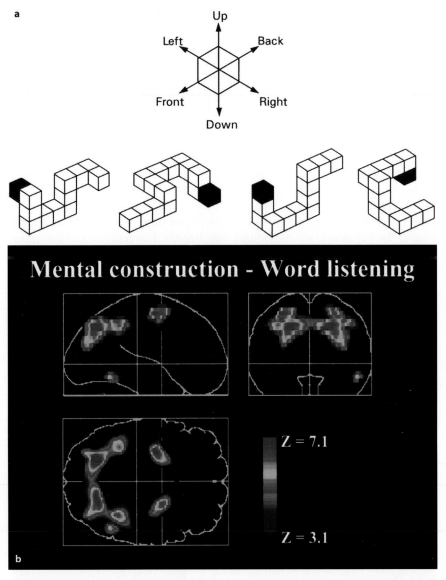

Fig. 4. *Functional anatomy of spatial visual imagery.* **a.** *Three-dimensional cube assemblies that a subject was asked to visualize during positron emission tomography to measure brain blood flow.* Thirty seconds before injection of ^{15}O-labeled water, a subject was asked to visualize a starting cube (gray) at the center of his field of view and to add cubes according to a list of 11 directional words binaurally delivered by earphones. **b.** *Lateral brain image of significant increments in blood flow during construction of cube assemblies versus listening to words without construction.* Mental construction activated the bilateral occipitoparietal-superior occipital cortex, inferior parietal cortex and premotor cortex and right inferior temporal cortex but not primary visual areas. Results show that the dorsal route known to process visuospatial features can be recruited by verbal without visual stimuli. Views of brain: left upper, sagittal; right upper, coronal; left lower, transverse. Z scores indicating statistical significance given on color bar (from Mellet et al. 1996)

Longevity Contributed to Brain Growth in Primates Through Natural Selection of Kinships

As originally proposed (Rapoport 1999), the scenario of Figure 2 ignored a possible contribution of longevity to natural selection in primates. Nevertheless, evidence of the importance of cooperation in primate kinships suggests that such a contribution can exist. If an extended unit of evolution were the kinship of genetically related individuals, an older individual, even if not himself reproductively successful, could nevertheless extend his genes in the general population by helping his kin to be competitive and reproduce (Hamilton 1964; Michod 1999; Mitteldorf and Wilson 2000; Wilson 1997). This longevity contribution is identified as the highlighted + in Figure 2.

A role in primate evolution of kinship units is consistent with evidence of cooperation among living primates in a variety of survival activities, sometimes even at the expense of an individual's own benefit. Cooperation can contribute to defense, hunting, food gathering, tool making, planning, child rearing, and migration (Jones et al. 1992; O'Connell et al. 1999). Indeed, a recent report in humans suggests that cooperative behavior is associated with activation of a region in the prefrontal association cortex (McCabe et al. 2001).

It is difficult to prove conclusively that cooperation was a positive fitness factor in promoting longevity during primate evolution. However, cooperation contributes to the survival of living hunter-gatherer tribes, in which older adults are more competent in hunting and tool making than are adolescents and young adults (Kaplan, this volume). Prolongation of a primate mother's life through the adolescence of her child can increase the likelihood of the child's survival (Clarke 1968; Kalin and Carnes 1984; Pryce et al. 1993), as can having experienced grandparents (O'Connell et al. 1999).

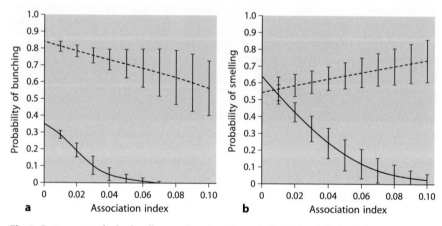

Fig. 5. *Responses to playback calls, as a function of association index (relationship) with caller, for families of African elephants directed by young matriarchs (mean age 35 years, dashed line) or old matriarchs (mean age 55 years, solid line).* Probabilities of (**A**) bunching or (**B**) smelling as defensive stress responses (from McComb et al. 2001)

A positive contribution of longevity to kin survival has been demonstrated in a long-lived nonprimate species, *Loxodonta africanus* (African elephant; Fig. 5; McComb et al. 2001). African elephant herds led by older compared with younger matriarchs are better able to distinguish known, friendly herds from unknown, potentially unfriendly herds, thus reducing the need for prolonged and stressful defensive actions. These superior "recognition" abilities correlate with a higher per capita reproductive success possibly because stress provoked spontaneous abortions and reduce fecundity in the females (Arck 2001; Kalin and Carnes 1984; Packer et al. 1995).

Conclusions

In the context of natural selection among individuals, prolongation of gestation, infancy, adolescence and young adulthood can easily be seen to be a positive fitness factor leading to more cognitively capable, larger-brained primate species. Prolonged gestation produces larger brains at birth, whereas prolonged maturation and young adulthood helps to maintain intense neuroplasticity so as allow ideation and cognition to enhance brain function in genotypes faced with new social and cognitive stresses.

It also is proposed that longevity was a positive fitness factor in primate evolution because the kinship as well as the individual was a unit of natural selection. Because of cooperation within kinships, larger-brained and more cognitively and socially capable older individuals could have enhanced the survival and reproductive success of their kin, thereby indirectly extending their own genes within the population. A recent study demonstrated this latter process for another long-lived species, the African elephant (McComb et al. 2001).

Acknowledgments

I thank Dr. Eugene Streicher for kindly reading and commenting on this paper.

References

Ameli NO (1980) Hemispherectomy for the treatment of epilepsy and behavior disturbance. Can J Neurol Sci 7: 33-38.
Arck PC (2001) Stress and pregnancy loss: role of immune mediators, hormones and neurotransmitters. Am J Reprod Immunol 46: 117–123.
Beck BB (1975) Primate tool behavior. In: Tuttle RH (ed), Socioecology and psychology of primates (Hawthorne NY, Mouton), p 575.
Beck H, Goussakov IV, Lie A, Helmstaedter C, Elger CE (2000) Synaptic plasticity in the human dentate gyrus. J Neurosci 20: 7080–7086.
Beckman KB, Ames BN (1998) The free radical theory of aging matures. Physiol Rev 78: 547–581.
Benowitz LI, Perrone-Bizzozero NI, Finklestein SP, Bird ED (1989) Localization of the growth-associated phosphoprotein GAP-43 (B-50, F1) in the human cerebral cortex. J Neurosci 9: 990–995.

Blest AD (1963) Longevity, palatability and natural section in five species of new world saturnid moth. Nature 197: 1183–1186.

Cabelli RJ, Hohn A, Shatz CJ (1995) Inhibition of ocular dominance column formation by infusion of NT-4/5 or BDNF. Science 267: 1662–1666.

Campbell BG (1988) Humankind emerging, 5th Ed. Glenview, Scott, Foresman and Co.

Campisi J (2000) Aging, chromatin, and food restriction – connecting the dots. Science 22: 2062–2063.

Cann RL, Stoneking M, Wilson AC (1987) Mitochondrial DNA and human evolution. Nature 325: 31–36.

Cantalupo C, Hopkins WD (2001) Asymmetric Broca's area in great apes. Nature 414: 505.

Changeux J-P (1983) L'Homme neuronal, Paris: Fayard.

Clarke AD (1968) Learning and human development. Brit J Psychiatr. 114: 1061–1077.

Constantine-Paton M (1990) NMDA receptor as a mediator of activity-dependent synaptogenesis in the developing brain. Cold Spring Harb or Symp Quant Biol 55: 431–443.

Corbetta M, Miezin FM, Dobmeyer S, Shulman GL, Petersen SE (1991) Selective and divided attention during visual discriminations of shape, color, and speed: Functional anatomy by positron emission tomography. J Neurosci 11: 2383–2402.

Darwin C (1871) The descent of man and selection in relation to sex, Vol 49, Princeton: Princeton University Press.

Darwin C (1859) The origin of species by means of natural selection London: Penguin Books.

Deacon TW (1992) The human brain. In: Jones S, Martin R, Pilbeam D (eds.) The Cambridge encyclopedia of human brain evolution, Cambridge: Cambridge University Press, pp. 115–123.

Dehay C, Giroud P, Berland M, Smart I, Kennedy H (1993) Modulation of the cell cycle contributes to the parcellation of the primate visual cortex. Nature 366: 464–466.

Dunbar R (1992 a) Social behavior and evolutionary theory. In: Jones S, Martin R, Pilbeam D (eds) The Cambridge encyclopedia of human evolution, Cambridge: Cambridge University Press, pp. 145–147.

Dunbar RIM (1992 b) Neocortex size as a constraint on group size in primates. J Human Evol 20: 469–493.

Feinberg I (1983) Schizophrenia: caused by a fault in programmed synaptic elimination during adolescence. J Psychiatr Res 17: 319–334.

Fischer RA (1958) The genetical theory of natural selection, Oxford: Clarendon Press.

Gallup Jr GG (1977) Self-recognition in primates. A comparative approach to the bidirectional properties of consciousness. Am Psychol 32: 329–338.

Gems D, Partridge L (2001) Insulin/IGF signalling and ageing: seeing the bigger picture. Curr Opin Genet Dev 11: 287–292.

Gould SJ (1977) Ontogeny and phylogeny Boston: Harvard University Press.

Gould E, Tanapat P, Rydel T, Hastings N (2000) Regulation of hippocampal neurogenesis in adulthood. Biol Psychiat 48: 715–720.

Hamilton WD (1964) The genetic evolution of social behaviour. I. J Theor et Biol 7: 1–52.

Harman D (1992) Free radical theory of aging. Mutation Res 275: 257–266.

Hatanpää K, Isaacs KR, Shirao T, Brady DR, Rapoport SI (1999) Loss of brain synaptic proteins regulating plasticity in human aging and Alzheimer's disease. J Neuropathol Exp Neurol 58: 637–643.

Hinke RM, Hu X, Stillman AE, Kim SG, Merkle H, Salmi R, Ugurbil K (1993) Functional magnetic resonance imaging of Broca's area during internal speech. NeuroReport 6: 675–678.

Hofman MA (1983 a) Encephalization in hominids: Evidence for the model of punctuationalism. Brain Behav Evol 22: 102–117.

Hofman MA (1983 b) Energy metabolism, brain size and longevity in mammals. Q Rev Biol 58: 495–512.

Hofman MA (1989) On the evolution and geometry of the brain in mammals. Prog Neurobiol 32: 137–158.

Holden C (1997) Overstimulated by early brain research? Science 278: 1569–1571.

Huttenlocher PR (1990) Morphometric study of human cerebral cortex development. Neuropsychologia 28: 517–527.

Huttenlocher PR (1979) Synaptic density in human frontal cortex – developmental changes and effects of aging. Brain Res 163: 195-205.

Huttenlocher PR, Dabholkar AS (1997) Developmental anatomy of prefrontal cortex. In: Krasnegor NA, Lyon GR, Goldman-Rakic PS (eds) Development of the prefrontal cortex: evolution, neurobiology and behavior, Baltimore: Paul H. Brookes, pp. 69-83.

Jones S, Martin R, Pilbeam D (1992) The Cambridge encyclopedia of human evolution, Cambridge: Cambridge University Press.

Kalin NH, Carnes M (1984) Biological correlates of attachment bond disruption in humans and non-human primates. Prog Neuropsychopharmacol Biol Psychiat 8: 459-469.

Kimura M (1983) The neutral theory of molecular evolution, Cambridge: Cambridge University Press.

Knipper M, Köpschall I, Rohbock K, Köpke AKE, Bonk I, Zimmermann U, Zenner H-P (1997) Transient expression of NMDA receptors during rearrangement of AMPA-receptor-expressing fibers in the developing inner ear. Cell Tissue Res 287: 23-41.

Kosslyn SM, Thompson WL, Kim IJ, Alpert NM (1995) Topographical representations of mental images in primary visual cortex. Nature 378: 496-498.

Kosslyn SM, Pascual-Leone A, Felician O, Camposano S, Keenan JP, Thompson WL, Ganis G, Sukel KE, Alpert NM (1999) The role of area 17 in visual imagery: convergent evidence from PET and rTMS. Science 284: 167-170.

Lovejoy CO (1981) The origin of man. Science 211: 341-350.

Martin GM (1996) Genetic modulation of the senescent phenotype of Homo sapiens. Exp Gerontol 31: 49-59.

Martin GM (2001) Frontiers of aging. Science 294: 13.

Martin RD (1990) Primate origins and evolution: a phylogenetic reconstruction, Princeton: Princeton University Press.

Matsuzawa T (1994) Field experiments on use of stone tools by chimpanzees in the wild. In: Wrangham RW, McGrew WC, De Waal FBM, Heltne PG (eds) Chimpanzee cultures, Cambridge: Harvard University Press, pp. 351-370.

McCabe K, Houser D, Ryan L, Smith V, Trouard T (2001) A functional imaging study of cooperation in two-person reciprocal exchange. Proc Natl Acad Sci USA 98: 11 832-11 835.

McComb K, Moss C, Durant SM, Baker L, Sayialel S (2001) Matriarchs as repositories of social knowledge in African elephants. Science 292: 491-494.

Medawar PB (1955) The definition and measurement of senescence. Ciba Found Colloq Ageing 1: 4-15.

Medawar PB, Medawar JS (1983) Aristotle to zoos. A philosophical dictionary of biology, Cambridge: Harvard University Press.

Mellet E, Tzourio N, Crivello F, Joliot M, Denis M, Mazoyer B (1996) Functional anatomy of spatial mental imagery generated from verbal instructions. J Neurosci 16: 6504-6512.

Melov S, Ravenscroft J, Malik S, Gill MS, Walker DW, Clayton PE, Wallace DC, Malfroy B, Doctrow SR, Lithgow GJ (2000) Extension of life-span with superoxide dismutase/catalase mimetics. Science 289: 1567-1569.

Michod RE (1999) Darwinian dynamics. Evolutionary transitions in fitness and individuality, Princeton: Princeton University Press.

Mitteldorf J, Wilson DS (2000) Population viscosity and the evolution of altruism. J Theor et Biol 204: 481-496.

Neve RL, Finch EA, Bird ED, Benowitz LI (1988) Growth-associated protein GAP-43 is expressed selectively in associative regions of the adult human brain. Proc Natl Acad Sci USA 85: 3638-3542.

Newport EL (1990) Maturational constraints on language learning. Cogn Sci 14: 11-28.

O'Connell JF, Hawkes K, Blurton Jones NG (1999) Grandmothering and the evolution of homo erectus. J Human Evol 36: 461-485.

Packer C, Collins DA, Sindimwo A, Goodall J (1995) Reproductive constraints on aggressive competition in female baboons. Nature 373: 60-63.

Pagel MD, Harvey PH (1988) How mammals produce large brained offspring. Evolution 42: 948-957.

Povinelli DJ, Eddy TJ (1996) Chimpanzees: joint visual attention. Psychol Sci 7: 129-135.

Pryce CR, Dobeli M, Martin RD (1993) Effects of sex steroids on maternal motivation in the common marmoset (Callithrix jacchus): development and application of an operant system with maternal reinforcement. J Comp Psychol 107: 99–115.

Puca AA, Daly MJ, Brewster SJ, Matise TC, Barrett J, Shea-Drinkwater M, Kang S, Joyce E, Nicoli J, Benson E, Kunkel LM, Perls T (2001) A genome-wide scan for linkage to human exceptional longevity identifies a locus on chromosome 4. Proc Natl Acad Sci USA 98: 10 505-10 508.

Rakic P (1988) Specification of cerebral cortical areas. Science 241: 170–176.

Rakic P, Bourgeois J-P, Eckenhoff MF, Zecevic N, Goldman-Rakic PS (1986) Concurrent overproduction of synapses in diverse regions of the primate cerebral cortex. Science 232: 232–235.

Rapoport SI (1990) Integrated phylogeny of the primate brain, with special reference to humans and their diseases. Brain Res Rev 15: 267–294.

Rapoport SI (1999) How did the human brain evolve? A proposal based on new evidence from in vivo brain imaging during attention and ideation. Brain Res Bull 50: 149–165.

Rasmussen DT, Izard MK (1988) Scaling of growth and life history traits relative to body size, brain size, and metabolic rate in lorises and galagos (Lorisidae, primates). Am J Phys Anthropol 75: 357–367.

Roland PE (1982) Cortical regulation of selective attention in man. A regional cerebral blood flow study. J Neurophysiol 48: 1059–1078.

Rumbaugh DM, Pate JL (1984). The evolution of cognition in primates: a comparative perspective. In: Roitblat HL, Bever TG, Rerrace HS (eds) Animal cognition, Hillsdale, N.J.: Lawrence Earlbaum Associateor, pp. 569–587.

Rumbaugh DM, Washburn DA, Hillix WA (1996) Respondents, operants and emergents: toward an integrated perspective on behavior. In: Pibram K, King J (eds) Learning as a self-organizing process, Hillsdale, NJ: Lawrence Earlbaum Associates, pp. 57–73.

Savage-Rumbaugh ES, Murphy J, Sevcik RA, Brakke KE, Williams SL, Rumbaugh DM (1993) Language comprehension in ape and child. Monographs Soc Res Child Develop 58: 1–254.

Sohal RS, Weindruch R (1996) Oxidative stress, caloric restriction, and aging. Science 273: 59–67.

Tomasello M, Call J (1997) Primate cognition Oxford: Oxford University Press.

Van Voorhies WA, Ward S (1999) Genetic and environmental conditions that increase longevity in Caenorhabditis elegans decrease metabolic rate. Proc Natl Acad Sci USA 96: 11 399–11 403.

Wallace DC (1992) Mitochondrial genetics: a paradigm for aging and degenerative diseases. Science 256: 628–632.

Whiten A, Goodall J, McGrew WC, Nishida T, Reynolds V, Sugiyama Y, Tutin CEG, Wrangham RW, Boesch C (1999) Cultures in chimpanzees. Nature 399: 682–685.

Wilson AC (1985) The molecular basis of evolution. Sci Am 253: 164–173.

Wilson DS (1997) Human groups as units of selection. Science 276: 1816–1817.

Educational level and longevity

J. F. Dartigues, L. Letenneur, C. Helmer, Ch. Lewden, G. Chêne

Summary

Educational level is known as a strong predictor of mortality before the age of 65. The relationships between education and early mortality from coronary heart disease, cancer and accidents consistently show an inverse pattern. More surprising is the association of mortality and education in AIDS patients.

The effect of education on early mortality has several interpretations; education is considered to be an indicator of socio-economic resources and a predictor of system integrity, healthy behaviours and entry to safer environments.

After the age of 65, the effect of education is less well known. With the Paquid cohort we have shown that educational level remains a risk factor for death, independently of cognitive decline or dementia.

Before the age of 65, inequalities in mortality related to socio-economic status are a generalised phenomenon in the industrialised world (Leclerc et al. 1990). In each country where data are available, death rates have been found to be higher in groups with lower occupational status, lower educational level, or lower income level (Kunst and Mackenbach 1994). However, the strength of the association between educational level and longevity is strongly related to the country of residence. Kunst and Mackenbach (1994) compared the death rates in men in several countries according to educational level (Table 1). In this analysis, inequalities were estimated by the proportional mortality increase moving from the top to the bottom of education. A total inequality estimate of 0.36 in subjects aged 55 years and older in Sweden, which is the lowest in this table, implies, according to the fitted regression equation, that death rates estimated for those at the bottom of the Swedish educational hierarchy are 36 % higher than the death rates estimated for those at the top. Inequalities in mortality are relatively small in the Netherlands and Scandinavia and more pronounced in the United States and France, while United Kingdom occupies intermediate position. The large inequalities in mortality in the US and France were attributed in part to large inequalities in education in these countries. Indeed, in the collaborative Eurodem study (Letenneur et al. 2000), the level of education appeared to be more variable in France than in the United Kingdom or the Netherlands. Thus the inequalities were larger in France and the power of the analysis to detect differences in mortality according to educational categories would be greater.

Finch et al. (Eds.)
Brain and Longevity
© Springer-Verlag Berlin Heidelberg 2003

Table 1. Mortality differences accociated with educational level among men by country and age group (Kunst and Mackenbach 1994)

Country	Total inequality estimate		
	35–44 years	45–54 years	55–64 years
Netherlands	0.72		
Denmark	1.17		
Norway	1.02		
Sweden	1.20	0.60	0.36
Finland	1.49	0.99	0.79
England	1.04	0.75	
France	1.97	1.59	1.28
Italy	1.85		
United States	2.62	1.06	1.05

Another important result of Kunst and Mackenbach was that, whatever the country, the inequalities in mortality related to education seemed to decrease with age. For instance, in France the total inequality estimate was of 1.97 in the younger age category, 1.59 in the middle and 1.28 in the older age category. This phenomenon could be related to a cohort effect, implying that the differences between higher and lower education were less pronounced in older people than in younger people, which would be a little bit surprising. A more rational explanation is that surviving people with low education were more resistant to disease than those who died in the younger age category. This heterogeneity in the population could explain why many risk factors linked to education do not have the same impact in a given disease according to age category.

Educational Level and Cause of Death

The relationships between educational level and early mortality from coronary heart disease, cancer and accidents consistently showed an inverse pattern. In a long-term follow-up of a cohort of 78,505 men born in 1932 and examined for military service in 1950–1951, Doornbos and Kromhout (1990) have shown that the risk of death decreased when the level of education increased, with the same magnitude in these three major causes of death before the age of 65. Interestingly, the association between total mortality and education remained unchanged after adjustment for such major risk factors for death as systolic blood pressure, heart rate, body-mass index, height or a cumulative health score. That means that education is related to survival independently of the exposure to these factors.

The same association exists for infectious disease. An interesting analysis was conducted in our INSERM Unit by Charlotte Lewden and Geneviève Chêne in Bordeaux on the relationship between educational level and mortality in the patients with Human Immuno-deficiency Virus (HIV) infection treated by protease inhibitors who constituted the multicentric APROCO cohort (Lewden 2001). In a univariate analysis, the educational level appeared to be a strong risk factor for death, with a relative risk of 4.8 for subjects with primary or second-

Table 2. Relationship between poor prognosis risk factors and educational level in patients with HIV infection. The APROCO study

Factors	University level	Primary/secondary
Transmission of HIV		
Homosexuality	56 %	32 %
Intravenous drugs	8 %	24 %
Anti-HCV antibodies	17 %	30 %
CD4 + mean	316	280
Unemployment	32 %	53 %
Married	59 %	51 %
Depression	42 %	54 %

ary level versus those of university level, and of 3.7 for subjects with no diploma. In fact, an analysis of the distribution of poor prognosis factors at the baseline screening showed that subjects with a low educational level cumulated almost all of these factors: higher frequency of subjects injecting intravenous drugs; more subjects with Hepatitis C antibodies, lower CD4 + lymphocytes count, lower proportion of married subjects, more unemployed subjects, and more depressed subjects (Table 2).

Surprisingly, after adjustments on all these factors, the association between education and death rate remained strongly significant, and even the relative risks increased to 6.4 and 8.2, respectively, for subjects with primary or secondary level education and subjects with no diploma. These findings could be related to multiple interactions between these poor prognosis factors. Educational level certainly represented the best social indicator of these interactions.

Indeed, the effect of education on mortality has several interpretations that are non-exclusive and provide a cumulative pejorative effect. Education is considered to be an indicator of socio-economic resources and a predictor of system integrity, healthy behaviours and entry to safer environments. Finally, education can also reflect the effect of multiple factors on the developing brain and can be an indicator of intelligence. Whalley and Deary (2001) recently underlined the impact of childhood Intelligence Quotient (IQ) on survival in a cohort of children from Aberdeen.

Education and Longevity in Elderly People

Education is not only a strong predictor of survival at 65 years of age, but also a strong predictor of successful ageing. In a recent paper, Vaillant and Mukamal (2001) defined successful ageing as being alive without permanent disability at a given age. They analysed the rates of permanent disability and death in two cohorts of men. The first one consisted of 237 Harvard sophomores (i.e., with a high level of education) selected for physical and mental health circa 1940. The second cohort consisted of 332 socially disadvantaged men from the core city of Boston. The rates of permanent disability and death were far higher in socially disadvantaged men, but the differences disappeared when one considered only the sub-sample of male college graduates in the core city cohort. Despite great differences in parental social class, prestige of college, intelligence test scores, income and job status, the health decline of the men from Boston who completed 16 or more years of education was no more rapid than that of Harvard sophomores. In other words, education may have been a more robust cause of the differences between the rate of health decline in the two cohorts than other differences in socio-economic status.

After the age of 65, the effect of education on mortality is less well known. The Paquid cohort was specifically designed to study brain and functional ageing in the south west of France (Dartigues et al. 1991). In this cohort, the educational level appears to be a predictor of mortality in elderly people, after controlling for age and gender. We estimated the relative risk of dying at 1.26 (95 % confidence interval = 1.12–1.43) after 10 years of follow-up of the cohort in subjects with no education or primary level education versus subjects with higher levels of education.

Since low education is recognised as a strong risk for dementia and Alzheimer's disease in this cohort (Letenneur et al. 1999), and since dementia is one of the major killers of elderly people (Helmer et al. 2001), a large part of the effect of education on longevity in elderly people could be attributed to dementia or cognitive decline. However, the inclusion of incident dementia as a time-dependent covariate in the model did not change the relationship between education and survival. Thus, the effect of education on longevity remains significant in elderly people and this effect seems to be independent of the effect of education on cognitive decline.

In conclusion, educational level appears to be one of the major determinants of longevity, whatever the age category.

References

Dartigues JF, Gagnon M, Michel P, Letenneur L, Commenges D, Barberger-Gateau P, Auriacombe S, Rigal B, Bedry R, Alpérovitch A, Orgogozo JM, Henry P, Loiseau P, Salamon R (1991) Le programme de recherche paquid sur l'épidémiologie de la démence. Méthodes et résultats initiaux. Rev Neurol 147: 225–230

Doornbos G, Kromhout D (1990) Educational level and mortality in a 32-year follow-up study of 18-year-old men in the Netherlands. Int J Epidemiol 19: 374–379

Helmer C, Joly P, Letenneur L, Commenges D, Dartigues J (2001) Mortality with dementia: results from a French prospective community-based cohort. Am J Epidemiol 154: 642–648

Kunst A, Mackenbach J (1994) The size of mortality differences associated with educational level in nine industrialized countries. Am J Public Health 84: 932–937

Leclerc A, Lert F, Fabien C (1990) Differential mortality: some comparisons between England and Wales, Finland and France, based on inequalities measures. Int. J Epidemiol 4: 1–10

Letenneur L, Gilleron V, Commenges D, Helmer C, Orgogozo J, Dartigues J (1999) Are sex and educational level independent predictors of dementia and Alzheimer's disease? Incidence data from the Paquid project. J Neurol Neurosurg Psychiat 66: 177–183

Letenneur L, Launer LJ, Andersen K, Dewey ME, Ott A, Copeland JRM, Dartigues JF, Kragh-Sorensen P, Baldereschi M, Brayne C, Lobo A, Martinez-Lage JM, Stijnen T, Hofman A (2000) Education and the risk for Alzheimer's disease: sex makes a difference. EURODEM pooled analyses. Am J Epidemiol 151: 1064–1071

Lewden C (2001) Facteurs associés à la mortalité dans une cohorte d'adultes infectés par le VIH-1 ayant débuté un traitement par inhibiteur de la protéase APROCO. Bordeaux, University Victor Ségalen, Bordeaux II.

Vaillant G, Mukamal K (2001) Successful aging. Am J Psych 158: 839–847

Whalley L, Deary I (2001) Longitudinal cohort study of childhood IQ and survival up to age 76. BMJ 322: 819–822

Incidence of Dementia Related to Medical, Psychological and Social Risk Factors: A Longitudinal Cohort Study During a 25-Year Period

G. Samuelsson[1], O. Dehlin[2], B. Hagberg[1], G. Sundström[3]

Abstract

This study is based on an entire cohort (n = 192) of 67-year-old persons born in 1902 and 1903 and living in a community in Southern Sweden. All subjects participated in interviews, psychological tests, and medical examinations. All contacts with primary health care and social services were recorded, as were death diagnoses. The cohort has been followed since 1969, with nine examinations until age 92.

The incidence rate (per 1000 person years) of dementia between 67 and 92 years of age, including those alive at age 92 as well as those deceased prior to 92, was 2.8 in the first five-year period, increasing up to 44.5 between ages 87 and 92. Altogether 16 % developed dementia during the period. The mean age for diagnoses of dementia was 80 years.

Fifteen presumptive social, medical and psychological risk factors for dementia have been applied (Cox regression analyses). Neither gender nor education were significant risk factors for dementia. Non-smokers tended to have a higher risk for dementia, but not a significantly higher risk. Normal blood pressure tended to increase the risk for dementia nearly significantly (p = 0.07). Diabetes increased the risk for dementia, however not significantly (p = 0.08). Using Cox regression analysis with dementia as a time-dependent covariate, it was found that dementia significantly increased the relative risk for death more than three times (CI 1.9–5.7), controlling for gender, smoking, diabetes, blood pressure, and education. Four cognitive tests were not found to be risk factors for dementia; neither were any of the medical parameters or social network variables.

Background

The purpose of the present study (the Dalby project) is to assess the incidence rate of dementia in a community-based cohort during a 25-year period and to relate dementia to medical, psychological and social characteristics at age 67.

[1] Gerontology Research Centre, Lund, Sweden
[2] Department of Community Medicine, Malmö, Sweden
[3] Institute of Gerontology, Jönköping, Sweden

Finch et al. (Eds.)
Brain and Longevity
© Springer-Verlag Berlin Heidelberg 2003

We are not aware of any other longitudinal study of this length that includes information about deceased persons and a range of multi-disciplinary predictors for dementia.

Incidence Studies

Among the few incidence studies with long follow-up, the Lundby study (Hagnell et al. 1990) found, during a 15-year period (age 60 and above), the risk for senile dementia of the Alzheimer type to be 25.7 % for men and 26.2 % for women. When only the very severely impaired were taken into account, the figures were 14.5 % in men and 14.6 % in women.

Prevalence Studies

Hofman et al. (1991) found that the overall European dementia prevalences from age 60 to 94 ranged between 1.0 and 32.2 %. Several Swedish studies have reported on prevalence for dementia. Skoog et al. (1993) reported a 21.4 % prevalence of dementia at 85 years of age for severe and moderate dementia and up to a 29.8 % prevalence when also mild forms of dementia were included. Johansson and Zarit (1995) found signs of mild, moderate and severe dementia in 19 % of a population at age 84. Adolfsson et al. (1981) reported a prevalence rate of 18.5 % at 85 years age, which is consistent with the Swedish OCTO study (Johansson and Zarit 1995). The H 70 study in Gothenburg (Nilsson 1984; Skoog 1993) reported similar prevalences. According to Fratiglioni (1993) the prevalence rate for the group 90+ in the Kungsholm study was 17 % for both men and women, with more than five times higher prevalence among women. Helmchen et al. (1999) found in the Berlin Aging Study that dementia affected 14 % of those aged 70 years and above and the corresponding figure for 90 year olds was 40 %. In a Swedish study of centenarians (Samuelsson et al., 1997) 27 % were diagnosed with dementia according to DSM III-R criteria. In comparison with other centenarian studies, the prevalence of dementia in the Swedish centenarian study was low. In a Japanese centenarian study, 68 % were reported to be demented (Homma et al. 1990), whereas 48 % were demented in the Hungarian centenarian sample (Beregi and Klinger, 1989). In a Finnish sample (Louhija 1994) the corresponding figure was 44 %. In general, prevalences for dementia are found to be quite heterogeneous, even in the same age groups.

Risk Factors for Dementia

Fratiglioni (1993) made an extensive literature review regarding *risk factors* for dementia. Including only studies with incidence data, she reported the following risk factors: age, female gender, manual occupation, non-smoking, and high alcohol consumption. However, the results were often contradictory. Vetter (1998) and Fratiglioni and Wang (2000) completed extensive reviews of smoking and Alzheimer's disease and reported that most epidemiological studies found a highly significant *negative* association between smoking and Alzheimer's disease. However, they pointed out that those results might have been affected by selective survival, and their own test of this "smoking protection hypothesis" failed to confirm it during the three-year follow-up (Fratiglioni and Wang 2000).

The risk of Alzheimer's disease has been consistently observed to be higher among individuals with little or no formal education, according to a literature review by Mayeux (1999). Low educational level was not found to be a risk factor for dementia in the Kungsholm study nor in the Swedish twin study (Gatz et al. 2001) but other studies have shown mixed results regarding education as a risk factor. Mayeux (1999) also found age and female gender to be risk factors for death among demented persons. A recent follow-up study over three years (Fratiglioni et al. 2000) found that poor quality of the social network increased the risk of dementia by 60 %. In the Lundby Study, precipitating as well as protective social and psychological factors for dementia of the Alzheimer type were studied (Hagnell et al. 1992). No social factors were found to be either precipitating or protective, whereas below average intelligence alone was a risk factor for men.

Samuelsson et al. (1994 a) found, regarding prediction of mental decline during a 13-year period, that the group with cognitive dysfunctions was characterized by low intelligence, more often single or still married, low degree of need satisfaction and low social class at age 67. Women suffering cognitive dysfunction were characterized by less anxiousness, higher social rigidity, more diseases at 67, and poor coping ability.

Reported medical risk factors for dementia included brain injures/head trauma (Mayeux 1999), arthritis, depression, and diabetes (Fratiglioni 1993). Guo (1998) found a cross-sectional relationship between relatively low blood pressure and dementia. According to Reisberg (1995) and Fratiglioni (2000), senile dementia was associated with a decrease in life expectancy. Also Agüero-Eklund (1998) and Helmer et al. (2001) found that dementia/Alzheimer's disorders were a major risk factor for reduced life expectancy even among the oldest old.

The *purpose* of the present study is:
1) To assess the incidence of dementia between ages 67 and 92 for all persons in the cohort under study;
2) To analyse medical, psychological and social risk factors for dementia over a 25-year period.
3) To study dementia as a risk factor for death

Materials and Methods

Population

The study population was based on one entire cohort (n = 192) of 67-year-old persons born in 1902 and 1903 and alive in June 1969 and June 1970. This population lived in the Dalby Primary Health Care District, close to Malmö, the third largest city in Sweden. The Dalby Primary Health Care center was the first in Sweden with training for medical students and research on the agenda.

Thirty-two persons refused participation and six men died prior to the examinations. However, we have collected information on mental diagnoses and formal care for the non-participants, as well as for the 12 persons who moved out of the health care district during the 25-year period. The non-participants had previously lived more often in urban than in rural areas. There were no differences between participants and non-participants in gender, marital status, mobility during earlier life or social class, although with regard to a more specific variable concerning economic level, non-participant men had a higher economic level than did those who participated; the opposite was true for women (Samuelsson et al. 1994 b).

Among the non-participants, 10.5 % had dementia diagnoses according to the health register. The dropouts may have been under-diagnosed during the observation period since they did not participate in the extensive follow-up examinations.

With regard to background factors for the participating group, the general level of education was approximately the same, or slightly lower, than in the corresponding age group for the country as a whole. The men had been primarily engaged in manual occupations (86 %) and the women (88 %) in household work or manual work, a typical pattern for a rural, turn-of-the-century cohort in Sweden. Two percent lived in old age homes at age 67 and the rest in the community. Fifteen percent were living alone. Males were clearly over-represented, also typical for older rural populations (Quensel 1945). All surviving persons except one participated in the follow-ups. The participation in the nine interview rounds varied between 72 % and 100 %; the latter includes survivors at age 92.

Methods

All subjects participated in an interview, psychological testing and an extensive medical examination at age 67. The sample has been followed since 1969 (from age 67) with repeated clinical examinations and interviews, normally every second year up to 1985 (at age 83). After that, one examination was made in 1994–95, when the group had reached age 92. All subjects have been followed until the age of 92 or until their death. Eighty-nine percent of the study group died between the ages of 67 and 92.

The interviews were completed by staff members attached to the project from the start. The accumulated information on each individual is extensive.

The medical and psychological data were collected at the local health care centre by a physician and a psychological team, and the examinations took approximately a day and a half to complete. The medical data, collected by a physician, included a full medical history of current and earlier diseases. Medical tests included complete blood tests, urine analysis, and ECG as part of the standard physical examination. Standardized psychological tests measured personality, cognition, needs, attitudes, adjustment, and included several intelligence tests (Samuelsson et al. 1994 b). Furthermore, all contacts with medical and social services were recorded as well as information from the death certificates. In addition, a social worker followed up with an in-home visit and interviewed subjects about their earlier and present life situations. This took approximately three hours. Findings from this study have been reported earlier (e.g., Hagberg et al. 1991); Samuelsson et al. 1993, 1994 a, 1994 b, 1998).

Social Measures

An interview questionnaire based on previous Swedish studies was used for the sociological investigation. Variables included in the present analysis are: occupation/social class, economic status, urban/rural and migration (during the life span), educational level, marital status, social networks, social support, child contact, and loneliness.

Social class was coded according to the Swedish SEI-coding system: self-employed (included farm owners and business owners), white collar and blue collar (Statistics Sweden, 1982). Information on economic status was obtained from assessed income from ages 65 to 68 years. Information regarding "Urban/Rural living" from birth to age 67 was collected from the population registry and subjects were classified accordingly. One group was classified as urban, one as rural, and the remainder were classified as mixed rural/urban living. Information concerning migration frequencies from birth to age 67 was collected from the population registry.

Loneliness was assessed on a four-point Likert scale and then dichotomized as 1) Never/Seldom or 2) Sometimes/Often. The attitude that time passes slowly was measured on a dichotomous scale: 1) Yes or 2) No.

Psychological Measures

The psychological examination covered personality measures, cognitive tests and a test of attitudes toward the future. The following tests were administered at age 67:
1) Cognition was assessed by a psychometric test battery that combined 14 tests measuring different aspects of logical inductive reasoning; verbal, numeric, and spatial abilities; intelligence; and motor speed (Lindberg et al. 1980). A previous factor analysis established factors that describe cognitive functions: ability to process theoretical knowledge, manual dexterity and speed, and perceptual and motor speed.

2) Indices of "Future view" and "Self concept" were based on attitude scales that measured participants' attitudes to different periods in their life as well as towards themselves (Samuelsson et al. 1994 b). "Future View" concerns whether the participants view the future in positive or negative terms.

Medical variables

The following was measured in the clinical examination: Cardiac disorders/symptoms, hypertension (diagnosed high blood pressure $> 160/90 = 1$, normal $= 2$, Diabetes Mellitus, dizziness, health at age 67 and earlier, medication: Sleeping pills, analgesics, sedative/hypnotic medication $(0) =$ no diseases or medication, $(2) =$ diseases or medication, smoking at age 67 or previous smoker $(1 =$ yes, $2 =$ no). Present Health (at age 67) measured the presence of the following disorders: diabetes mellitus, rheumatoid arthritis, angina pectoris, lung disease, gastrointestinal disease, liver disease, kidney disease, or cancer, and then recorded on a dichotomous scale: 1) $=$ No diseases or 2) $=$ One or more diseases.

In addition to the extensive medical examinations, primary health care data about mental diagnoses as well as date of death have been collected for all persons, including those who died before age 92. Persons with suspected dementia symptoms were examined by a geriatrician. Diagnostic classification systems have changed since 1969. During the period 1969 to 1977, "The Provisional Diagnosis Codes for Open Care" (The National Board of Social Welfare 1970), which were built on ICD 8, were used as a classifications system for mental disorders at the Primary Care Center in Dalby. During the period 1978 to 1986, "Diagnosis Codes in Open Care" were used (The National Board of Social Welfare 1977). Since 1987, the International Classification of Health Problems in Primary Care 2 (ICHPPC-2-Defined; 1986) was used. Dementia, in general, was defined, based on all available data, according to DSM-III and no attempt was made to differentiate into the various forms of dementia (Alzheimer's disease, vascular dementia, frontal lobe dementia).

Other sources of information were records from home health care and nursing homes. For the group who died between ages 83 and 92, managers of old age homes and nursing homes and case managers in Home Help services answered questions about suspected dementia disorders among their clients. Later controls of the medical journals was made of this group. The thorough knowledge of the persons' health histories improved the diagnostic validity of dementia. Incidence rates of dementia were calculated for the entire 25-year period and in five-year periods.

Statistical Analysis

The Pearson Chi-Square test was used to test relationships between two categorial variables. Cox regression analyses was used to assess risk factors for dementia. Cox regression with dementia as a time-dependent covariate was used to analyse risk factors for early death.

Results

Social and Psychological Characteristics of Non-Demented and Demented Persons

Table 1 shows the social and psychological characteristics at base line for non-demented persons and for those who became demented. Only for gender was there any significant difference; females more often developed dementia. The variable rural/urban living (during the whole life span up to age 67) showed a nearly significant difference; rural living was more frequent among persons who developed dementia. Length of education, economic status, marital status, having children or loneliness did not show any significant differences between

Table 1. Social and psychological characteristics at base line for non-demented and those who developed dementia (column percent, and mean values)

Social variables	Non-demented (n = 129)[a]	Demented (n = 25)[b]	P-value
Gender (%)			
Male	62.8	40.0	0.03[c]
Female	37.2	60.0	
Taxed income (%)			
Low	61.1	41.7	NS
High	38.9	58.3	
Education, years			
Mean	7.2	6.9	NS
Rural/urban living (%)			
Rural	67.4	87.5	0.11
Mixed rural/urban	24.8	12.5	
Urban	7.8	–	
Marital status (%)			
Single	20.2	20.0	NS
Married	71.3	68.0	
Widowed/divorced	8.5	12.0	
Children (%)			
Yes	25.8	20.0	NS
No	74.2	80.0	
Loneliness (%)			
Never/seldom	80.0	79.2	NS
Often/sometimes	20.0	20.8	
Psychological variables (means)			
Theoretical function	4.8	5.3	NS
Problem solving	5.0	5.3	NS
Motor skill	4.8	5.3	NS
Knowledge	4.9	5.3	NS
Positive future view	4.9	6.0	0.03[c]

[a] N varied between 122 and 129
[b] N varied between 21 and 25
[c] *:P < 0.05

demented and non-demented persons; neither did social class, network variables or social contact variables (not shown in the table). The four cognitive tests did not show any significant differences. However, looking at the trends in the four tests, those who eventually developed dementia had the highest scores on all four tests. Regarding the test "Positive attitude to the future," persons diagnosed with dementia were significantly more often positive about the future.

Medical Characteristics of Non-Demented and Demented Persons

Smoking at or before age 67 was not a risk factor for dementia but the reverse; smokers were less likely to have dementia (Table 2). Physician visits before age 67 was nearly significant; demented person had made more visits. None of the medical variables – blood pressure, diabetes, health at age 67, heart symptoms – was significantly related to dementia development; neither was medication (sleeping pills, pain medication, tranquilizer medicine).

Table 2: Medical characteristics at base line for non-demented and demented persons (column percent, and mean values)

	Non-demented	Demented	P
Blood pressure (%)			
Not normal	27.6	20.8	NS
Normal	72.4	79.2	
Diabetes (%)			
No	96.1	91.3	NS
Yes	3.9	8.7	
Present health (%)			
No problems	60.2	52.2	NS
Some problems	39.8	47.8	
Doctor visits before 67 (%)			
No visits	49.2	30.4	0.09
Visits	50.8	69.6	
Heart problems (%)			
No symptoms	91.5	95.7	NS
Some problems	8.5	4.3	
Smoker, present or earlier (%)			
Yes	44.5	20.8	0.03[a]
No	55.5	79.2	

[a] *:P < 0.05

Incidence of Dementia During the 25-Year Period

Figure 1 shows the incidence of dementia per 1000 person years in five-year periods from ages 67 to 92. The incidence rate was 2.8 in the first period, increasing up to 17.5 at age 82 to 87. During the last period, between age 87 and 92, the incidence rate for the survivors was 44.5.

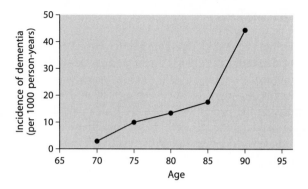

Fig. 1. Incidence of dementia
per 1000 person-years

Risk Factors for Dementia

Table 3 shows the relative risk of dementia of the five strongest variables from the bivariate Cox regression analyses of 15 presumptive social, medical and psychological base line variables. Neither gender nor education was a significant risk factor for dementia. Non-smokers had a higher risk of dementia, though not significant. Normal blood pressure increased the risk of dementia nearly significantly (P = 0.07). We also tested the risk of dementia with more differentiated groupings of blood pressure (quartiles of blood pressure). Results from these analyses did not show any increase or decrease in risks of dementia. Diabetes increased the risk for dementia, however not significantly (p = 0.08).

Table 3. Relative risks of dementia (RR) with 95 % confidence interval estimated from a Cox regression model

Risk factors	RR	95 % CI	P
Gender (1 = male, 2 = female)	1.3	(0.42– 4.2)	0.63
Education (years)	0.84	(0.56– 1.3)	0.42
Smoker (1 = yes, 2 = no)	1.9	(0.49– 7.1)	0.36
Blood pressure (1 = high 160/90, 2 = normal)	3.2	(0.91–11.2)	0.07
Diabetes (1 = no, 2 = yes)	3.7	(0.84–16.3)	0.08

Dementia and Survival

Using Cox regression analysis (with dementia estimate dependent covariate) we found that dementia significantly increased the relative risk for death more than three times (3.3) (CI 1.9–5.7, P < 0005). The analysis was performed controlling for gender, smoking, diabetes, blood pressure, and education (years).

Discussion

Using all persons in a community-based cohort, we investigated the incidence of dementia during a 25-year period, as well as risk factors for dementia. The incidence rate per 1000 person years was 2.8 in the first five-year period, increasing up to 44.5 between ages 87 and 92. The total risk to develop dementia during the period was 16%. The mean age for onset of dementia was 80 years. Bivariate analyses with base line characteristics showed that females, non-smokers and persons with positive future attitudes were significantly more often diagnosed with dementia. Controlling for confounding variables of selective survival, these variables were not significant risk factors.

Dementia diagnosis increased the relative risk for death more than three times. Our study did not show any significant predictive value for social network variables for dementia; neither did the four cognitive tests.

Among the very few incidence studies with long follow-up the Lundby study (Hagnell et al. 1992) showed the risk of senile dementia of the Alzheimer type to be 25.7% for men and 26.2% for women during a 15-year period. When only the very severely impaired were taken into account, the figures were 14.5 in men and 14.6 in women. These results are in reasonable agreement with the present ones. Comparing our results to prevalence studies, Skoog et al. (1993) reported a 21.4% prevalence of dementia at 85 years of age for severe and moderate dementia. Our findings are similar to Johansson and Zarit (1995), who found signs of mild and severe dementia in 18% of a population at the age of 84 years, and by Adolfsson et al. (1981), who reported a prevalence rate of 18.5% for 85 year olds. According to Fratiglioni (1993), the prevalence rate for the group 90+ in the Kungsholm study was 17% for both genders (17.6 in our study) with a more than five times higher prevalence among women.

How can we interpret the results from the *risk factor analyses*? Neither gender nor education was a significant risk factor for dementia in this study, in contrast to what was found in several other studies. Low educational level was not a risk factor for dementia in the Kungsholm five-year follow-up study (Fratiglioni 1993) or in the Gatz et al. (2001) Swedish twin study.

Diabetes increased the risk for dementia, though not significantly ($p = 0.08$). This finding might be explained by compliance with medication among demented persons. Normal blood pressure increased the risk for dementia nearly significantly ($P = 0.07$). Regarding blood pressure we further tested the risk with more differentiated groupings of blood pressure (quartiles of blood pressure). These analyses did not result in any significant increased or decreased risks for dementia. Yet, Guo (1998) found a cross-sectional relationship between relatively low blood pressure and dementia.

Non-smokers had a higher risk (Cox regression) for dementia; however, not a significantly higher risk. Vetter (1998) and Fratiglioni and Wang (2000) reported in extensive reviews of smoking and Alzheimer's disease that most epidemiological studies found a highly significant *negative* association between smoking and Alzheimer's disease. However, they pointed out that those results might be an effect of selective survival. Fratiglioni and Wang (2000) failed to confirm the smoking protecting hypotheses.

None of the social network variables – marital status, contact variables, and loneliness – were related to dementia development. Our study does support the findings of Fratiglioni et al. (2000), as neither study finds a significant predictive value of the *quantitative* network variables for dementia. However, they found a significant relationship between *qualitative* network aspects and dementia progress.

A dementia diagnosis increased the relative risk for death more than three times. This finding has been confirmed in several studies (Mayeux 1999).

Our study has both weaknesses and strengths. One *weakness* is that the results are based on a relatively small population that gives relatively low power in statistical analyses. Furthermore, many of our base line predictors may change during the 25-year period, such as the network variables, marital status, and medical and psychological variables (not social class, education). When interpreting the results, one must bear in mind that such changes during the period might influence the risk factor pattern.

A *strength* of our study is that it includes all persons in a local cohort, with information on non-participants, the institutionalized and the deceased. The number of drop-outs during the follow-up period is very low (one person). Extensive multidisciplinary examinations have been completed and information from medical and social records has been collected. We have not found any other study with the same length of follow-up period of one specific community-based cohort. To compare our results with the results from other prevalence and incidence studies of dementia might thus be problematic. During the period 1969 to the middle of the 80s, doctors were probably less prone to diagnose dementia because expertise and knowledge was partly lacking. However, as the study group participated in intensive examinations every second year and had check-ups of suspected dementia by specialists, the diagnoses during this period are probably more sensitive. During the period 1984 (when the group was 82 years old) to 1994, the awareness and knowledge of dementia among doctors were higher than before. Thus, the diagnosis for the deceased between ages 84 and 92 might be of fairly good quality.

In conclusion, our incidence rate seems to be in line with several of the prevalence studies as well as with the few incidence studies. Our results from the risk factor analyses for dementia are both contradictory and supportive of other studies.

Acknowledgements

This study was supported financially by the Delegation for Social Research (grant DSF 88 37 : 1) and the Ribbing Memorial Foundation. Vibeke Horstmann provided help in the statistical analysis and valuable criticism. Professor of Geriatrics Lars Gustafson completed a control of all persons suspected of having dementia between age 67 and age 83. Cheryl McCamish-Svensson assisted with English corrections.

References

Adolfsson R, Gottfries CG, Nyström L, Winblad B (1981) Prevalence of dementia disorders in institutionalized Swedish old people. The work load imposed by caring for these patients. Acta Psych Scand 63: 225–244.

Agüero-Eklund H (1998) Natural history of Alzheimer's disease and other dementias. Findings from a population survey. Academic Dissertation. Karolinska Institute, Stockholm.

Beregi E, Klinger A (1989) Health and living conditions of centenarians in Hungary. Int Psychogeriatrics 1: 195–200.

Fratiglioni L (1993) Epidemiology of Alzheimer's disease, Academic Dissertation. Acta Neurol Scand Munksgaard Copenhagen, 145: 87.

Fratiglioni L, Wang H-X (2000) Smoking and Parkinson's and Alzheimer's disease: review of the epidemiological studies. Behav Brain Res 113: 117–120.

Fratiglioni L, Wang H-X, Ericsson K, Maytan M, Windlad B (2000) Influence of social network on incidence of dementia: a community-based longitudinal study. The Lancet 355: 1315–1319.

Gatz M, Svedberg P, Pedersen NL, Mortimer JA, Berg S, Johansson B (2001) Education and the risk of Alzheimer's Disease: findings from the study of dementia in Swedish twins. J G Psych Sci 56 B (No 5): P 292–300.

Guo Z (1998) Blood pressure and dementia in the very old. An epidemiologic study. Academic Dissertation, Karolinska Institute, Stockholm.

Hagberg B, Samuelsson G, Lindberg B, Dehlin O (1991) Stability and change of personality in old age and its relation to survival. J Gerontol Psych Sci 6: 285–291.

Hagnell O, Essen-Möller E, Lanke J, Öjesjö L, Rorsman B (1990) The incidence of mental illness over a quarter of a century. Almqvist and Wiksell International, Stockholm.

Hagnell O, Frank A, Gräsbeck A, Öhman R, Otterbeck L, Rorsman B (1992) Senile dementia of the Alzheimer type in the Lundby Study. Eur Arch Psychiat Clin Neurosci, 241: 231–235.

Helmchen H, Baltes MM, Geiselmann B, Kanowski S, Linden M, Reischies FM, Wagner M, Wernicke T, Wilms H-U (1999) Psychiatric illnesses in old age. In: Baltes PB, Mayer KU (eds) The Berlin aging study. Aging from 70 to 100. Cambridge University Press, Cambridge, 167–175.

Helmer C, Joly L, Lettenneur D, Commenges D, Dartigues J-F (2001) Mortality with dementia: results from a French prospective community-based cohort. Am J Epidemol, 154: 642–648.

Hofman A, Rocca WA, Brayne C, Breteler MM, Clarke M, Cooper B, Copeland JRM, Dartigues JF, Da Silva Droux A, Hagnell O, Heeren TJ, Engedahl K, Jonker C, Lindesay J, Lobo A, Mann AH, Mölsä PK, Morgan K, O'Connor DW, Sulkava R, Kay DWK, Amaducci L (1991) For the Eurodem prevalence research group. The prevalence of dementia in Europa. A collaborative study of 1980–1990 findings. Int J Epidemiol 3: 736–748.

Homma A, Nakazato K, Shimonaka Y (1990) Centenarians in Japan. A gerontopsychiatric survey. In: Hasegawa K, Homma K (eds) Psychogeriatrics Biol Soc Adv Exerpta Medica Amsterdam, Princetown, 351–356.

Johansson B, Zarit S (1995) Prevalence and incidence of dementia in the oldest old: a longitudinal study of a population-based sample of 84–90-year-olds in Sweden. Int J Geriat Psychiat 10: 359–366.

Lindberg B, Nordén Å, Nyberg P, Samuelsson G (1980) Var älder har sin fördel, Studentlitteratur, Lund.

Louhija J (1994) Finnish centenarians, A clinical epidemiological study. Academic Dissertation, University of Helsinki, Helsinki.

Mayeux R (1999) Predicting who will develop Alzheimers disease. Mayeux R, Christen (eds) Epidemiology of Alzheimers disease: from gene to prevention. Fondation Ipsen, Paris.

National Board of Health and Social Welfare (1970) Provisional diagnosis codes for open care.

National Board of Social Welfare (1977) Diagnosis codes in open care.
National Board of Social Welfare (1986) International classification of health problems in primary care 2.
Nilsson L-V, Persson G (1984) Prevalence of mental disorders in an urban sample examined at 70, 75 and 79 years of age. Acta Psych Scand 69: 519–527.
Quensel CE (1945) Befolkningsförhållanden i Sverige. Statistiska undersökningar kring befolkningsfrågan. SOU 1945: 53.
Reisberg B (1995) Senile dementia. In: Maddox GL (ed) The encyclopedia of aging. Second Edition. Springer Publishing Company. New York.
Samuelsson G, Dehlin O, Rundgren Å (1993) Differences in health status and mortality in an urban and rural populations – effects of long-term exposure. Intl J Health Sci 1: 3–12.
Samuelsson G, Hagberg B, Dehlin O (1994 a) Retirement status predicting health conditions 16 years later. Ageing Soc 14: 29–52.
Samuelsson G, Hagberg B, Dehlin O, Lindberg B (1994 b) Medical, social and psychological factors as predictors of survival – a follow up from 67 to 87 years of age, Arch Gerontol Geriatr 18: 25–41.
Samuelsson S-M, Bauer Alfredson B, Hagberg B, Nordbeck B, Samuelsson G, Brun A, Gustafson L, Risberg J, Robertsson E (1997) The Swedish centenarian study – physical and mental health. Aging human devel 45: 223–253.
Samuelsson G, Andersson L, Hagberg B (1998) Loneliness in relation to social, psychological and medical variables over a 13 period – a study of elderly in a Swedish rural district. J Mental Health Aging 3: 320–327.
Skoog I, Nilsson L, Palmertz B, Andreasson L-A, Svanborg A (1993) A population-based study of dementia in 85-year-olds. New Engl Med 3: 153–158.
Statistics Sweden National Central Bureau of Statistics. Liber, Stockholm.
Vetter JN (1998) Smoking. In: Pathy MSJ (ed) Principles and practice of geriatric medicine, Third Edition. John Wiley & Sons, Ltd., London.

Cognitive Impairment and Survival at Older Ages

H. Maier[1], M. McGue[2], J. W. Vaupel[1, 3], K. Christensen[3]

Summary

Several studies have suggested that cognitive impairment is a risk factor for mortality among older adults. However, the mechanisms that generate the association between cognitive function and survival are not well understood. Proposals attempting to explain why the association is observed focus on the role of health and diseases and on terminal decline. Poor health may affect both cognitive function and survival, and the association between cognitive impairment and mortality could be spurious. The terminal decline hypothesis suggests that factors related to the death of the individual cause a decline in intellectual performance, and that the onset of this decline may be detected in some instances several years prior to the death of the persons.

We investigated these issues in a sample of 2,401 Danish twins aged 75 years and older. At baseline in 1995 the Mini-Mental State Exam was administered to assess participants' cognitive functioning, and subjective and objective health measures were also collected. We related cognitive function to six-year survival. As expected, cognitive impairment was associated with an increased risk of death. Interestingly, this effect was attenuated but not eliminated after statistical controls for a number of health measures, suggesting that the association between cognitive function and survival is robust and can only in part be attributed to health factors.

A second set of analyses addressed the terminal decline hypothesis. Surviving participants were re-contacted and re-interviewed in 1997 and 1999. A total of 984 individuals participated in all three waves. Consistent with the terminal decline hypothesis, there was evidence that decline in cognitive function was more pronounced among in those who died when compared to the survivors. However, a history of cognitive decline did not predict mortality above and beyond the current level of cognitive functioning.

[1] Max Planck Institute for Demographic Research, Rostock, Germany.
[2] Department of Psychology, University of Minnesota, Minneapolis, USA.
[3] Institute of Public Health, University of Southern Denmark, Odense, Denmark.

Finch et al. (Eds.)
Brain and Longevity
© Springer-Verlag Berlin Heidelberg 2003

Introduction

With aging, both "normal" senescent, age-related changes and late-onset diseases may affect the brain, producing declines in performance and resulting in
mild or severe cognitive impairment. In contemporary industrialized societies,
approximately 5 to 10 % of the population aged more than 65 years suffers from
dementia. Milder cognitive dysfunction is estimated to be at least two times as
prevalent (Graham et al. 1997). Cognitive impairment represents a major public
health burden with adverse psychosocial and economic consequences for the
affected persons and their families. There are also a number of research reports
suggesting that cognitive impairment predicts subsequent mortality (for
reviews see Berg 1996; Siegler 1975; Small and Bäckman 1999).

Understanding the pattern in determinants of late-life survival becomes
increasingly important as the population ages (Christensen and Vaupel 1996).
However, the mechanisms that generate the association between cognitive
impairment and mortality are not well understood. It has often been speculated
that the association arises as a consequence of other factors. In the present
study we examined two groups of potentially confounding covariates: indicators
of socioeconomic status and indicators of health. Persons with higher socioeconomic status tend to live longer (Kitagawa and Hauser 1973). It is also known
that socioeconomic status and cognitive function are correlated (Lindenberger
and Baltes 1997), and the observed association between cognitive function and
survival could be due to the higher socioeconomic status of those with higher
cognitive scores.

A similar argument has been made for health factors (Small and Bäckman
1999). Morbidity has an impact on cognitive performance (van Boxtel et al.
1998) as well as on mortality. Thus the association between cognitive impairment and mortality could be spurious, perhaps due entirely to health factors. In
the context of the present study, we had access to several health measures and
we explored whether inclusion of these measures would attenuate or even eliminate the association between cognitive function and survival.

It has also been argued that it is not the level of cognitive function that is
important when it comes to mortality and survival, but rather change and
decline in function. Specifically, it could be that the cognitive status is much less
important than a trajectory or history of decline. Kleemeier (1962) proposed
the so-called terminal decline hypothesis, which is still widely entertained
today. The hypothesis suggests "that factors related to the death of the individual cause a decline in intellectual performance, and that the onset of this decline
may be detected in some instances several years prior to the death of the person" (Kleemeier 1962, p. 293). If this were the case, then we would expect that
every sample of older persons includes a number of individuals in their terminal decline phase and, consequently, associations between baseline cognitive
function and mortality risk would be observed. Convincing empirical demonstration of terminal decline has remained somewhat elusive, because it is very
difficult to separate death-related changes from normative age-related decre-

ments in cognitive function. It is also unclear whether most or all people are eventually affected by terminal decline. It could be that only subgroups are susceptible to death-related decline in function, such as people with Alzheimer's disease. In the context of the present study we first explored whether terminal decline was present in a sample of persons aged 75 years and older. In a second step we investigated whether a history of decline was associated with mortality, above and beyond the current level of cognitive function.

Data and Methods

Study Population and Sample

Our data came from the Longitudinal Study of Aging Danish Twins (Christensen et al. 1999), a population-based Danish twin study. In March 1995 a survey was conducted among all Danish twins who were 75 years or older. Among the 3,099 individuals in the study population, extensive interview information was obtained on 2,401 individuals, corresponding to a participation rate of 77%. Interviews were conducted at the twins' residences. When a twin was unable to participate due to physical or mental handicaps, a proxy-responder was sought (closest relative). A total of 2,188 interviews were conducted with twins, and 213 interviews were conducted with proxies.

In 1997 and again in 1999, the surviving participants were re-contacted and the survey was repeated. A total of 1,595 twins (81% of the surviving 1995 participants) were re-interviewed in the 1997 wave; 984 twins (74% of the surviving two-wave participants) were re-interviewed in the 1999 wave.

Measure of Cognitive Impairment

The Mini-Mental State Examination (MMSE; Folstein et al. 1975) was used to assess cognitive impairment. The MMSE is a short interviewer-administered test including brief measures of calculation, language, orientation, recall and registration, with scores ranging from 0 to 30. For the purpose of the present analyses, scores on the MMSE were graded into four levels (high normal, low normal, mild impairment, severe impairment). Cutoffs for these levels are reported in the first column of Table 1. The chosen cutoffs are consistent with recommendations in the literature (e.g., McDowell and Newell 1996).

Measures of Socioeconomic Status

Two measures of socioeconomic status were employed. Elementary education was chosen as a measure reflecting socioeconomic status early in life. For the purpose of the present analyses, elementary education was graded into three levels: less than 7th grade, 7th–8th grade, and 9th grade and above. Social class was chosen as a measure of socioeconomic status in late life. Twins and their spouses were assigned to one of five social classes (Christensen et al. 1998; Hansen 1984). Twins were assigned to the social status of their spouse (alive or deceased) if it was higher than their own. For the purpose of the present analyses, social class was graded into two levels. The two highest social classes were collapsed into the level "high social class;" the three lowest social classes were collapsed into the level "low social class."

Health Measures

Three measures of health were employed. The number of hospitalizations from 1977 to 1994 was used as an externally assessed measure of general health. The National Danish Discharge Registry comprises information on practically all discharges from somatic hospitals in Denmark. Hospital information was obtained for all but 123 of twins through register linkage (Christensen et al. 1999). The present study was based on hospitalization of the twins in the period from January 1, 1977, through December 31, 1994. The number of hospitalizations was graded into four levels ("0," "1 to 2," "3 to 5," and "6 or more" hospitalizations).

A composite measure of functional abilities was selected to measure each person's functional health status. The composite measure reflects physical strength; it is based on self-reports and comprises 11 items focusing on mobility and the ability to walk, run, climb stairs and carry weights (Christensen et al. 2000). For the purpose of the present analyses, scores of the composite measure were divided into four levels according to quarters of the performance distribution ($< 25^{th}$ percentile; $\geq 25^{th}$ and $< 50^{th}$ percentile; $\geq 50^{th}$ and $< 75^{th}$ percentile; $\geq 75^{th}$ percentile).

A single-item subjective health measure was used to assess self-rated health. Participants were asked, "Do you think that your health is generally excellent, good, acceptable, poor, or very poor?" For the purpose of the present analyses, participants' responses were divided into four levels ("excellent," "good," "acceptable," and "poor or very poor" health).

Missing Values

Researchers studying cognitive function in older adults typically encounter a sizeable portion of missing data. It is unlikely that this type of missing data occurs at random. In dealing with missing values researchers have applied strategies such as listwise deletion or imputation of estimated values based on regression models. We chose a different approach with the goal of obtaining an estimate of the mortality risk associated with incomplete data on the MMSE. Specifically, for the MMSE and for other risk factor we included an additional level composed of the persons with missing data on that factor. Inspection of the relative risk associated with missing MMSE provides an estimate of the degree to which incomplete data on the MMSE are related to mortality. Anstey et al. (2001) reported that having incomplete cognitive and sensory data was associated with an elevated mortality risk in persons aged 70 and older, suggesting that missing data are predictive of subsequent mortality. Consequently, we expected that persons with missing MMSE data would have an increased mortality risk when compared to persons with complete data.

Mortality Follow-up

Mortality follow-up for all participants was conducted through register linkage with the Civil Registration System. A total of 1154 individuals (48.1 % of those with interview information in 1995) had died as of January 1, 2001, and their dates of death were recorded.

Procedure and Statistical Model

Cox proportional hazards regression models (Cox 1972) were evaluated for the effects of risk factors. We used the PHREG procedure (Allison 1995) from the SAS software package to estimate Cox regression models.

Results

Level of Cognitive Impairment and Survival

A first analysis focused on the bivariate association between level of cognitive impairment and mortality. From Model 1 in Table 1 it can be seen that the risk of death increased monotonically with decreasing level of cognitive function. Interestingly, those without an exam had the highest risk. These are the persons who participated by proxy or refused to take the MMSE. Their mortality risk was more than five times higher when compared to persons who scored in the "high normal" range.

We then inspected the relative risks obtained from a series of hierarchical models to gain insights into the pattern of association between cognitive impairment and mortality. Model 2 in Table 1 included statistical controls for age and sex. This adjustment reduced the relative risks associated with levels of cognitive impairment by about 20 to 25 %. Model 3 in Table 1 also controlled for two measures reflecting socioeconomic status early and late in life (elementary education and social class, respectively). Relative risks associated with levels of cognitive impairment remained virtually unaltered, indicating the association between cognitive function and survival cannot be attributed to level of elementary education or social class.

In a next step we asked whether the association remains after controls for three health measures (hospitalizations between 1977 and 1994, functional abil-

Table 1. Percentages and number of people who died until 2001, by level of cognitive impairment, and association of cognitive impairment with mortality among a sample of 2,401 persons who participated in the Longitudinal Study of Aging Danish Twins in 1995

| Mini-Mental State Exam | Total no. | Persons who died | | Relative risk adjusted for | | | | | | | |
| | | No. | % | Unadjusted (Model 1)[a] | | Age and sex (Model 2)[b] | | Age, sex, and SES (Model 3)[c] | | Age, sex, SES, and health (Model 4)[d] | |
				RR	95 % CI	RR	95 % CI	RR	95 % CI	RR	95 % CI
High normal (28–30)	637	198	31.1	1		1		1		1	
Low normal (24–27)	844	339	40.2	1.38	1.16, 1.64*	1.27	1.07, 1.52*	1.29	1.08, 1.53*	1.11	0.93, 1.33
Mild impairment (18–23)	494	276	55.9	2.23	1.86, 2.68*	1.84	1.53, 2.22*	1.86	1.54, 2.26*	1.35	1.11, 1.65*
Severe impairment (<18)	186	140	75.3	3.77	3.03, 4.68*	2.92	2.34, 3.65*	2.96	2.35, 3.73*	1.71	1.35, 2.18*
Missing	240	201	83.8	5.65	4.63, 6.88*	4.70	3.84, 5.77*	4.70	3.79, 5.83*	1.67	0.96, 2.89

[a] Relative risks were obtained from a Cox regression model including the Mini-Mental State Exam. RR, relative risk; CI, confidence interval

[b] Relative risks were obtained from a Cox regression model including the Mini-Mental State exam, age at interview, and sex

[c] Relative risks were obtained from a Cox regression model including the Mini-Mental State exam, age at interview, sex, elementary education, and social class (SES)

[d] Relative risks were obtained from a Cox regression model including the Mini-Mental State exam, age at interview, sex, elementary education, social class, hospitalizations from 1977–1994, functional abilities, and self-rated health

* p < .01

ities, and self-rated health). Adjustment for health measures reduced the relative risk by more than one half. It seems, then, that health factors are quite important when it comes to explaining the relation between cognitive function and mortality. However, it is noteworthy that even after adjustment for these health factors, cognitive impairment was still related to mortality, although the association was less pronounced.

In a final step we explored whether there were age and sex differences in the predictive pattern. We addressed this question by including interaction terms (age group × MMSE; sex × MMSE) in the regression model. Neither the interaction involving age group (ages 75–84 versus ages 85+) nor the interaction involving sex reached statistical significance. Thus it appears that the association between cognitive impairment and survival is similar for ages 75–84 and ages 85+, as well as for women and men.

It is known that genetic influences on cognitive function are substantial (McGue and Christensen 2001). There is also evidence that genetic factors affect length of life (Herskind et al. 1996; McGue et al. 1993). The analyses presented above included a sub-sample of n = 480 intact twin pairs and this sub-sample may have affected our estimates of the association between cognitive function and survival. We examined this issue in a set of separate analyses relying exclusively on unrelated twins. Specifically, for this set of analyses we randomly selected and omitted one twin from each intact twin pair. The relative risks obtained among 1,920 unrelated twins were very similar to relative risks observed in the full sample, suggesting that the inclusion of persons who share all or half of their genes did not artificially inflate the reported relative risks.

Terminal Decline

We investigated patterns of terminal decline among 984 twins who participated in the first three waves of the Longitudinal Study of Aging Danish twins in 1995, 1997, and 1999. Complete data on the MMSE were available for 858 twins. A total of 126 persons (12.8 % of the three-wave participants) had missing MMSE data at one or more measurement occasions; these persons were not considered in the longitudinal analyses.

In a first step, we examined average MMSE performance separately for those who survived (n = 755) and those who died (n = 103) prior to January 2001. Figure 1 displays their average MMSE scores in 1995, 1997, and 1999. On average, there was some decline for both survivors and the deceased. However, the average decline in cognitive function was much more pronounced in those who died before the year 2001. This pattern fits well with the terminal decline hypothesis: there was modest decline in the survivors, but much steeper decline in those who were near to death.

In a next step we moved from average performance to individual trajectories. We inspected plots of individual trajectories with the goal of finding out whether there were clear-cut differences between the trajectories of the survi-

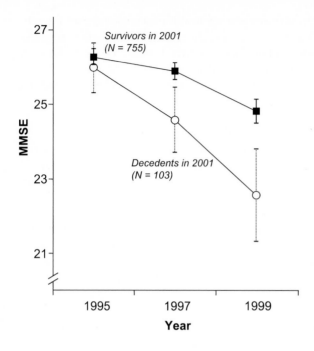

Fig. 1. Average MMSE score and 95 % confidence interval by year and vital status in 2001 among 858 persons who participated in the first three waves of the Longitudinal Study of Aging Danish Twins from 1995 to 1999

vors as compared to those of the deceased. Figure 2 shows a plot of 50 randomly selected trajectories from the survivors and 50 randomly selected trajectories from the deceased. The trajectories of the survivors and the deceased did not differ in an obvious way. Rather it appears that trajectories reflecting decline, maintenance, and even increase in cognitive function were present in both groups. This finding suggests that there were large inter-individual differences in intra-individual change among both survivors and the deceased.

When it comes to the prediction of mortality, is it sufficient to know a person's cognitive status or does information about the person's change in cognitive function improve the prediction? To address this question, we tried to summarize the slope of each twin's trajectory by a simple measure. Using data stemming from three measurement occasions it is possible in principle to investigate curvilinear patterns of change. However, we restricted our attention to a linear model of change, which is less dependent on chance fluctuations in the data. For each twin we calculated an average MMSE gain measure, obtained as the slope parameter of a linear regression of MMSE score on time-in-study (in years). Thus the MMSE gain measure reflects the individual's average rate-of-change in MMSE per year for the period from 1995 to 1999. We then used the MMSE gain measure to predict short-term mortality up to January 2001.

The MMSE gain measure was related to mortality risk (see Table 2). For every MMSE point gained per year, the mortality risk was lowered by 26 %. Or, conversely, for every MMSE point lost per year, the risk of death was increased by 26 %. This result remained unaltered when we statistically controlled for the

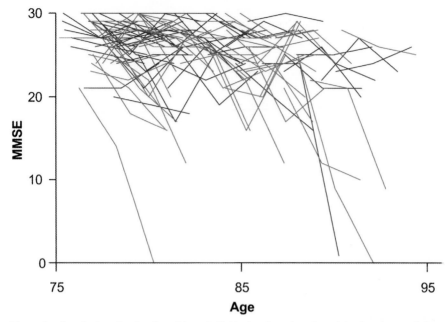

Fig. 2. One hundred randomly selected intra-individual trajectories of cognitive function. Each line denotes the trajectory of a person. Survivors are shown in blue, the deceased in red

initial MMSE level in 1995, suggesting that decline in cognitive function was associated with mortality above and beyond initial level of function.

We then applied a harder test to assess the role of change in the prediction of mortality, involving adjustment for final MMSE level in 1999. This analysis was designed to investigate whether a history of decline in cognitive function is predictive of mortality above and beyond the current level of functioning. From Table 2 it can be seen that the final MMSE level in 1999 was associated with short-term mortality. Addition of the MMSE gain measure did not significantly improve the prediction ($\chi^2 = 1.1$, df = 1, p > 0.05). However, it should be noted that the final MMSE level in 1999 and MMSE gain were highly correlated (r = 0.77, p < .01). That is, individuals who experienced large declines in MMSE were also highly likely to score low at the final MMSE assessment. Thus it was very hard for MMSE gain to predict mortality beyond final assessment, despite the evidence for terminal decline (cf. Fig. 1). Nevertheless, the analysis presented in Table 2 suggests that a history of decline in cognitive function was not associated with mortality above and beyond the current level of functioning. In sum, there was evidence that terminal decline in cognitive function occurred in some of the twins. Current level of cognitive function was associated with subsequent mortality, but a history of decline did not add to the prediction.

Table 2. Mortality risk until 2001 associated with initial MMSE in 1995, final MMSE in 1999, and change in MMSE among a sample of 858 persons who participated in the first three waves of the Longitudinal Study of Aging Danish Twins from 1995 to 1999

Risk factor	Unadjusted[a]		Change and initial level[b]		Change and final level[c]	
	RR	95 % CI	RR	95 % CI	RR	95 % CI
MMSE gain per year 1995–1999	0.74	0.65, 0.85*	0.74	0.65, 0.85*	0.87	0.68, 1.13
Initial MMSE in 1995	0.97	0.92, 1.03	0.96	0.91, 1.02		
Final MMSE in 1999	0.93	0.91, 0.96*			0.96	0.91, 1.01

Note. RR = relative risk; CI = confidence interval
[a] Unadjusted relative risks were obtained from a separate Cox regression model for each risk factor, that is, excluding other factors. RR, relative risk; CI, confidence interval
[b] Relative risks were obtained from a Cox regression model including MMSE gain per year 1995–1999 and initial MMSE in 1995
[c] Relative risks were obtained from a Cox regression model including MMSE gain per year 1995–1999 and final MMSE in 1999
* $p < .01$

Discussion

A number of recent research reports implicated higher levels of cognitive function as a predictor of survival (Anstey et al. 2001; Bassuk et al. 2000; Bosworth et al. 1999; Maier and Smith 1999; Neale et al. 2001; Smits et al. 1999; Whalley and Deary 2001). The present study replicated this finding in a sample of old and very old Danish twins. The Mini-Mental State exam was included as a screen for cognitive impairment with clinically relevant cutoffs. With decreasing level of cognitive function, mortality risk increased considerably. For example, individuals who were classified as severely impaired had a more than three times higher risk of dying compared to those who scored in the high normal range. A sizeable portion of this effect can be attributed to other known risk factors, such as age and health status. After statistical controls for these other factors, the effects of cognitive impairment were reduced in their magnitude. However, it is noteworthy that cognitive function remained a significant and sizeable predictor of survival even after adjustments for these other factors.

Incomplete data on the MMSE were associated with a substantially increased risk of death. It seems likely that incomplete data are indicative of very poor cognitive function. In the present study, 89 % of missing data on the MMSE occurred because some twins were unable to participate due to physical or mental handicaps and proxy responders were sought. Thus it is probably the case that the true association between cognitive function and survival is even more pronounced than was reported here.

There are several proposals in the literature attempting to explain why an association between cognitive function and survival is observed. Results from the present study suggest that the role of socioeconomic factors is negligible.

We do not wish to dispute the importance of socioeconomic factors – they are clearly important with respect to inequalities in health and survival (Marmot et al. 1995). However, the association between cognitive impairment and mortality can probably not be attributed to individual differences in socioeconomic factors.

An alternative explanation for the link between cognitive function and survival focuses on the role of health. Physical health may affect both cognitive function and mortality (Berg 1996), and the association between cognitive function and survival could be spurious. The present study lends some support to this proposal. Adjustment for three measures of health reduced the relative mortality risks associated with levels of cognitive function by more than one half. This finding suggests that the association can in part be attributed to health factors, although the etiologic mechanism remains to be specified.

Extensive and fine-grained models for measuring health status have been proposed (e.g., Idler 1992). It could be argued that controls for participants' health were not extensive enough in the present study, because only three measures of health were included. But then, the measures of health that were included were strongly related to survival, and nevertheless they did not eliminate the association between cognitive impairment and mortality. Moreover, in older adults chronological age is itself a substantial carrier of additional health information, and the link between cognitive function and survival was evident even after controls for both age and health measures. Thus, results from the present study suggest that cognitive function does make a difference in terms of survival, regardless of health. This conclusion is consistent with evidence from other studies that controlled for a large array of health measures (Smits et al. 1999) and physician-observed ICD diagnoses of illnesses (Maier and Smith, 1999).

If socioeconomic and health factors cannot fully account for the link between cognitive impairment and mortality, why do we observe this association? It is possible that cognitive impairment results in maladaptive everyday behavior, which in turn may increase an individual's risk of death. Everyday adaptive capacity comprises a large set of everyday behaviors, practices, and routines, which are directly or indirectly related to health and, ultimately, to survival. For example, it is adaptive to keep health care appointments, remember to take necessary medication, maintain sound preventive care and nutrition, recognize signs and symptoms of disease, seek timely medical assistance, operate electronic devices according to instructions, obey traffic rules, and so forth. Cognitive impairment may compromise an individual's everyday adaptive capacity in many ways, thereby increasing the susceptibility to death from a variety of causes.

Many researchers have recognized that behavioral adaptations may mediate the relation between cognitive function and survival (Bosworth et al. 1999; Swan et al. 1995). It would be interesting to know how much of the effect of cognitive function on survival is mediated through everyday behavioral adaptations. Unfortunately, it is very difficult to address this question empirically, because a comprehensive measure of everyday adaptive capacity has yet to be established. Some studies of cognition and mortality have included a small set of health practices, such as smoking status or alcohol consumption (e.g., Bassuk et al. 2000; Swan et al. 1995). Health practices did not emerge as prominent mediators of the effect of cognition on survival. However, the true effect of behavioral adaptations was probably severely underestimated in these studies, because only few and select aspects of everyday adaptive capacity were measured.

Cognitive function appears to be a marker of the human organism's capacity to survive. It has often been suggested that terminal decline can account for some or all of this. In the present study we undertook several longitudinal analyses with the goal of clarifying the relationship of terminal decline to mortality. Analyses comparing survivors and the deceased indicated a pattern consistent with the notion of terminal decline. On average, there was minor decline in the survivors and accelerated decline in the deceased. Inspection of individual trajectories, however, suggested that there is considerable inter-individual variability in patterns of cognitive decline. Among all persons who were near to death, it appeared that some experienced terminal decline while others did not. Future research should seek to determine the factors that characterize those who experience terminal decline. In this context it might be interesting to examine whether terminal decline is more prevalent among certain causes of death, such as Alzheimer's disease, cardiac disease, or stroke.

Cognitive decline was associated with higher mortality in this sample of Danish twins aged 75 years and older. Does cognitive decline confer an increased mortality risk above and beyond the level of functioning? This question is probably best addressed by choosing the resulting level of functioning as a comparison standard. We found that a history of cognitive decline did not confer an added mortality risk beyond the resulting level of function. That is, although there was evidence for terminal decline in this study, the decline per se did not signal an unfavorable prognosis not accounted for by the current level of functioning.

Conclusion

In a sample of Danish twins aged 75 and older, cognitive impairment was an independent predictor of six-year mortality after statistical controls for age, sex, measures of socioeconomic status, and measures of health. Effects appeared to be similar in women and men, as well as for ages 75–84 and ages 85+. Incomplete data on the cognitive measure were associated with a substantially increased risk of death. There was evidence that terminal decline in cognitive function was present among those who died. However, a history of decline did not predict mortality above and beyond current level of functioning.

Acknowledgment

The Longitudinal Study of Aging Danish Twins is supported by the U.S. National Institute on Aging research grant NIA-P01-AG08761 and the Danish National Research Foundation. Data are available for other researchers. Please see http://www.pubpol.duke.edu/centers/ppa/index.html for details.

References

Allison PD (1995) Survival analysis using the SAS system: a practical guide. SAS Institute Inc, Cary

Anstey KJ, Luszcz MA, Giles LC, Andrews GR (2001) Demographic, health, cognitive, and sensory variables as predictors of mortality in very old adults. Psychol Aging 16: 3–11

Bassuk SS, Wypij D, Bergman LF (2000) Cognitive impairment and mortality in community-dwelling elderly. Am J Epidemiol 151: 676–688

Berg S (1996) Aging, behavior, and terminal decline. In: Birren JE, Schaie KW (eds) Handbook of the psychology of aging. 4th Ed. Academic Press, New York, pp. 323–337

Bosworth HB, Schaie KW, Willis SL (1999) Cognitive and sociodemographic risk factors for mortality in the Seattle Longitudinal Study. J Gerontol B-Psychol 54: P272–P282

Christensen K, Vaupel JW (1996) Determinants of longevity: genetic, environmental, and medical factors. J Intern Med 240: 333–341

Christensen K, Gaist D, Jeune B, Vaupel JW (1998) A tooth per child? Lancet 352: 204

Christensen K, Holm NV, McGue M, Corder L, Vaupel JW (1999) A Danish population-based twin study on general health in the elderly. J Aging Health 11: 49–69

Christensen K, McGue M, Yashin A, Iachine I, Holm NV, Vaupel JW (2000) Genetic and environmental influences on functional abilities among Danish twins aged 75 years and older. J Gerontol A-Biol 55: M446–M452

Cox DR (1972) Regression models and life tables (with discussion). J Roy Stat Soc B 34: 187–220

Folstein MF, Folstein SE, McHugh PR (1975) "Mini-Mental State": a practical method for grading the cognitive state of patients for the clinician. J Psychiat Res 12: 189–198

Graham JE, Rockwood K, Beattie BL, Eastwood R, Gauthier S, Tuokko H, McDowell I (1997) Prevalence and severity of cognitive impairment with and without dementia in an elderly population. Lancet 349: 1793–1796

Hansen EJ (1984) Socialgrupper i Danmark. Socialforskninginstitutet, Copenhagen

Herskind AM, McGue M, Holm NV, Sorensen TIA, Harvald B, Vaupel JW (1996) The heritability of human longevity: a population-based study of 2872 Danish twin pairs born 1870–1900. Human Genet 97: 319–323

Idler EL (1992) Self-assessed health and mortality: A review of studies. In: Maes S, Leventhal H, Johnston M (eds) International Review of Health Psychology. Wiley, New York, pp. 33–54

Kleemeier R (1962) Intellectual changes in the senium. Proceedings of the Social Statistics Section of the American Statistical Association 1: 290–295

Kitagawa EM, Hauser PM (1973) Differential mortality in the United States: a study in socioeconomic epidemiology. Harvard University Press, Cambridge

Lindenberger U, Baltes PB (1997) Intellectual functioning in old and very old age: cross-sectional results from the Berlin Aging Study. Psychol Aging 12: 410–432

Maier H, Smith J (1999) Psychological predictors of mortality in old age. J Gerontol B-Psychol 54: P44–P54

Marmot M, Bobak M, Davey Smith G (1995) Explanations for social inequalities in health. In: Amick BC, Levine S, Tarlov AR, Walsh D (eds) Society and health. Oxford University Press, New York, pp. 172–210

McDowell I, Newell C (1996) Measuring health: a guide to rating scales and questionnaires. Oxford University Press, New York

McGue M, Christensen K (2001) The heritability of cognitive functioning in very old adults: evidence from Danish twins aged 75 years and older. Psychol Aging 16: 272–280.

McGue M, Vaupel JW, Holm N, Harvald B (1993) Longevity is moderately heritable in a sample of Danish twins born 1870–1880. J Gerontol 48: B237–B244

Neale R, Brayne C, Johnson AL (2001) Cognition and survival: an exploration in a large multicentre study of the population aged 65 years and over. Int J Epidemiol 30: 1383–1388

Siegler IC (1975) The terminal drop hypothesis: Fact or artifact? Exp Aging Res 1: 169–185

Small BJ, Bäckman L (1999) Time to death and cognitive performance. Curr Dir Psychol Sci 8: 168–172

Smits CHM, Deeg DJH, Kriegsman DMW, Schmand B (1999) Cognitive functioning and health as determinants of mortality in an older population. Am J Epidemiol 150: 978–986

Swan GE, Carmelli D, LaRue A (1995) Performance on the digit symbol substitution test and 5-year mortality in the Western Collaborative Group Study. Am J Epidemiol 141: 32–40

Van Boxtel MP, Buntinx F, Houx PJ, Metsemakers JF, Knotterus A, Jolles J (1998) The relation between morbidity and cognitive performance in a normal aging population. J Gerontol A-Biol 53: M147–M154

Whalley LJ, Deary IJ (2001) Longitudinal cohort study of childhood IQ and survival up to age 76. Brit Med J 322: 819–822.

What Do We Know About the Cognitive Status of Supercentenarians?

J. M. Robine[1] and *C. Jagger*[2]

Studies of the prevalence of dementia and of cognitive impairment have consistently shown a steady increase with age. The first models supported an exponential trajectory above the age of 65 years (Preston 1986; Jorm et al. 1987), suggesting that by the age of around 98 years all surviving persons would have dementia. These models were based on meta-analyses of prevalence studies conducted before the 1990s, and most prevalence studies of that time included few subjects who were nonagenarians or centenarians. A later meta-analysis (Ritchie et al. 1992) resulted in a model that increased the age at which all survivors would have dementia to 103 years.

At present, all we can surmise about the prevalence of dementia or cognitive impairment at advanced ages is based on the extrapolation of models fitted essentially to empirical data from 65 to 85 years of age. Above the age of 85 years, the confidence interval of the prevalence rate would be large enough to support any trajectory. Some authors have challenged that an exponential trajectory reasonably summarizes the experience of cognitive decline among the oldest old. The same arguments used in the study of mortality trajectories among the oldest old led to alternatives such as a logistic trajectory which would tend toward but never reach a ceiling of mortality (Thatcher 1999), or even a quadratic trajectory where the mortality rate would decline after some maximum value (Vaupel et al. 1998). Fitted to cognitive decline, the logistic trajectory will leave a proportion of the oldest old free from any significant cognitive decline (Ritchie and Kildea 1995) and the quadratic trajectory will lead to a decline in cognitive impairment after some maximum value, the rationale for such a trajectory being a combination of both the heterogeneity of the population, with some individuals being at higher risk of cognitive decline, and the selection brought by the mortality process.

Before the age of 100 years, these trajectories are not sufficiently differentiated to allow any empirical verification of the relationship between age and cognitive decline in the population. However, above the age of 100 years, they become progressively distinct, first the logistic and quadratic trajectories from

[1] INSERM, Université de Montpellier 1, Val d'aurelle, Parc Euromédecine, 34298 Montpellier cedex 5, France
[2] University of Leicester, Department of Epidemiology and Public Health, 22–28 Princess Road West, LEI 6TP Leicester, United Kingdom

Finch et al. (Eds.)
Brain and Longevity
© Springer-Verlag Berlin Heidelberg 2003

the exponential one, then the logistic from the quadratic trajectory. To suggest which trajectory might summarize cognitive decline in the oldest old, we will consider the cognitive status of the few persons to reach the age of 115, at present the farthest possible point after the assumed point of inflexion of about 85 years for the logistic or quadratic trajectories. Such people are "supercentenarians," defined as persons having reached at least the age of 110, with the first validated cases appearing in the 1960s with steadily increasing numbers since 1980 (Robine and Vaupel 2001). Hence if most people reaching the age of 115 show significant cognitive decline, this supports the exponential trajectory. If, however, they have a prevalence of cognitive decline similar to that of centenarians, this supports the logistic trajectory. Finally, if they manifest a prevalence of cognitive decline lower than that of centenarians, the quadratic trajectory is supported.

Several studies have already examined, at least partially, the cognitive status of centenarians. In 1990, the Ipsen Foundation undertook a piece of research entitled *"In search of the secret of the centenarians"* (Allard 1991). One of the goals was to examine the relationship between longevity and cognitive function. Eight hundred (800) centenarians were examined in 1990 and were followed until the year 2000. The Short Portable Mental Status Exam (SPMSE) of Pfeiffer was used to detect possible cases of dementia with a threshold of four errors or more, the same threshold as has been used in the younger elderly (Pfeiffer 1975). Thirty-five percent of the women examined and 55 % of the men (37 % of both sexes) made less than three errors at the screening test and were therefore classified as not having dementia. The remaining 63 % were classified as having dementia or had been unable to undergo the test because of sensory impairments or other reasons (Fondation Ipsen 1991; Allard and Robine 2000). International studies have confirmed the French results, although with different methods and tests. In Denmark, the percentage is identical: 37 % of the centenarians examined in 1995–1996 did not have signs of dementia according to the Mini Mental State Examination (MMSE; Andersen-Ranberg et al. 2001). In New England (USA) 36 % of the centenarians examined in 1997 were not suspected to have dementia (Silver et al. 2001). In Japan again 37 % of the centenarians examined in 1987–1989 were not suspected to have dementia (57 % of the men and 29 % of the women), and in Sweden, the results were even better for the centenarians examined between 1987 and 1992, with only 37 % of the centenarians classified as mildly, moderately, or severely demented according to the *DSM-III-R criteria*[1] (Hagberg et al. 2001).

Despite the variety of screening instruments and sampling methods, all the studies confirm that a substantial proportion of centenarians, between 35 and 40 %, appear to be free of dementia. This bracket is confirmed by a recent review of the literature dealing with other centenarian studies (Dewey and Copeland 2001). Thus, dementia appears not to be inevitable at the oldest ages.

---

[1] *Diagnostic and Statistical Manual of Mental Disorders* (*DSM-III-R*;American Psychiatric Association, 1987)

With regard to differences between the sexes, the prevalence of dementia has always been higher for women that men. All the studies dealing of centenarians, including the earliest ones in Hungary (Beregi and Klinger 1989) and Finland (Louhija 1994), confirm that the prevalence of dementia is still much greater among centenarian women than men. This finding can be explained in part by the greater survival with dementia of women over men. But educational differences between the sexes, a feature particularly of the older cohorts, may also contribute. We are now beginning to understand the effect of education on the level of cognitive performance and thus on the level of disability of the oldest old of today (Freedman et al. 2001; Robine et al. 2002). However, even if current results do not confirm the assumption of a levelling off of the prevalence of dementia for the highest ages (Ritchie and Kildea 1995), all epidemiological studies on the health status of centenarians show that a considerable proportion of them are free of dementia. Thus we are some way from the catastrophic scenarios predicted (Preston 1986; Jorm et al, 1987; Balansjaar et al., 2000) and indeed we may move further from these scenarios with the replacement of the older cohorts by the more recent ones who have higher levels of education and more experience with activities having strong cognitive input.

The Ipsen centenarian study was undertaken because of the unexpected rise in the number of centenarians observed in France in the 1980s. We now know that the number of centenarians has roughly doubled in France every ten years since 1950 (Vaupel and Jeune 1995) and that this Centenarian Doubling Time is shortening. Recently an international database on longevity – the IDL database – has been established to monitor the emergence of supercentenarians, persons having reached at least the age of 110 years (Robine and Vaupel, 2002). Two hundred and fifty eight (258) cases have already been gathered including a fairly complete list of 179 well validated cases corresponding to nine low mortality countries: Belgium, Denmark, England & Wales, Finland, France, Japan, Netherlands, Norway and Sweden.

But what do we know about the cognitive functioning of these extremely old people? How many are still free of dementia or is dementia inevitable at such advanced ages? It is very difficult to evaluate the cognitive status of supercentenarians with traditional approaches and screening tests developed for younger elderly (Ritchie 1995). For example, A.D., former farmer, did not remember the date of the day, the month, the season or even the year when he was 110 years old. He was unable to subtract 7 from 20 (basic elements of any screening test) but he was still able to have a meaningful conversation with his daughter, his nurses or his doctor. However, he kept the ability to ask for news about friends, family members and relatives and to show socially valued emotion until his death, if we exclude the last 10 days.

To study the cognitive status of supercentenarians, we decided to focus on this notion of meaningful conversation and to limit the study to the seven persons who had recently reached or surpassed the age of 115: six women and one man, whose ages were carefully validated. To evaluate their cognitive functioning during the last years of their life, we decided, with the collaboration of the researchers who had validated their ages, to contact their general practitioner and/or nursing home to ascertain when the last meaningful conversation took place. We asked first to what age the supercentenarian lived independently at home and the age at which they entered a nursing home or equivalent. Secondly, we asked when the last meaningful conversation had occurred with the supercentenarian, specifying that by meaningful conversation we meant a specific exchange with a personal/emotional/intellectual/or social content implying judgment. The exchange had to be specific and pertinent. For example a remark about a new dress or someone's appearance, such as, "You look pretty today," or "I like your dress," or a remark about a special day, "It is Christmas next week and I am happy (sad) . . ." We asked informants to exclude automatic, basic messages about activities of daily living, such as, "I want to go to the toilet," without any specific content, and inappropriate remarks, such as, "I want to go back and live at home," in their evaluation of the time of the last meaningful exchange. Then we reviewed, case by case, the cognitive status of the seven supercentenarians on the IDL database who had reached the age of 115: C.H., who died in England in 1993 aged 115; J.C., who died in France in 1997 at the age of 122; C.M., who died in California in 1998 at the age of 115; M.L.M., who died in Canada in 1998 at the age of 117; S.K., who died in the United States in 1999 aged 119; A.J., who died in England in 1999 aged 115; and M.B., who died in France in 2001 at the age of 115.

C.H. lived in the community until the age of 114, living alone until 112. She flew the Atlantic in the Concorde in a wheelchair for her 110th birthday and met the mayor of New York. C.H. remained mentally alert until her death at the age of 115, according to her close circle. Her ambition was to live to 120 (Laslett, personal communication).

J.C. lived alone until the age of 110, when she entered a nursing home. She remained totally independent until 114 when she broke her hip a few days before her 115th birthday (Robine and Allard 1998, 1999; Ritchie 1995). She remained mentally alert until the last week of her life, according to her doctor, when she was 122 years old.

C.M. lived in the community until 1978 when he was 96 years old, and then he entered a retirement community where he eventually died 20 years later, aged 115. Until about the age of 115 he was still capable of intelligent conversation, as demonstrated by the records of conversations kept by the researchers who investigated his case. At the last meeting about one week before his death, he was confused and delirious (Wilmoth et al. 1996). The principal investigator noted that all the conversations with C.M. were very slow and underlined that there were good and bad days. (This last remark was also made about the case of J.C., with days where it was easy to communicate with her despite her hearing impairments and days when these impairments seemed to prevent any useful conversation. In the case of M.B., presented later, the nursing home staff used to say, "she has her days . . .")

M.L.N. lived with her husband in the community until his death in 1972 when she was 92 years old, after which she lived with her daughter. She entered a nursing home in 1988 at the age of 107 (Desjardins 1999). According to her doctor, M.L.M. was completely demented at the end of her life (Desjardins, personal communication). On the occasion of her 117th birthday, journalists wrote, "As for Marie-Louise, today she does not speak much, but when she does, she can be pretty humorous;" remembering two years previously when her relatives sang "Happy Birthday" to her when she turned 115, she sang "Happy birthday to me." When they told her she was the oldest living Canadian she said, "Poor Canada." The press cuttings related to M.L.M. are typical of the newspaper cuttings concerning centenarians with low cognitive functioning: no direct interview, but the recall of a few pertinent comments. We will find the same type of information about M.B.

S.K. lived independently at home until the age of 100. She entered a nursing home at the age of 110 (Rodgers Mayer 1997). She was able to hold meaningful conversations until the age of 119. In December 1999, the day S.K. died, when K., her daughter was ready to go home after a visit, S.K. said, "Do you have to leave now?" K. said she had to go because the driver was waiting. S.K. said, "You tell him to take good care of you." Of course K. cherishes those last words of her mother's. Isn't it wonderful to be 98 and still have your mother trying to take care of you? K., who herself will be 100 this year, regularly plays bridge and often wins and her cognitive status appears excellent. K says that the above exchange was not typical of her mother's last six months; that she had been "vague" for about six months and not really responsive in conversation. However, prior to that (at age 118) she had had real conversations asking K how she was and what she had been doing. She would also ask "what was going on with the family?" and about specific members: "Tell me about Bob (her grandson)" (Sylver, personal communication).

A.J. lived at home until her death but had help to care for her. At 108 she still attended the 8.30 am church service on Sunday. At 110 she had a fall, was admitted to hospital and was then physically, although not mentally, incapacitated. She had a stroke around her 115th birthday. Our informant (A.B.) had a conversation with her around the time of her 114th birthday. A.J. was certainly in full possession of all her cognitive functions at that time, and our informant gave us two examples of this. She said to the wife of our informant: "I hope you are looking after him properly because if not I have a couple of bedrooms free and the garden needs doing!" A.B. also asked her if she had had a birthday card from the bishop. She replied "I had a card from someone called Jonathon with a cross beside the name – so it was either the bishop or a secret admirer." (Note: Anglican bishops use their first name and then a cross as a signature; Jagger, personal communication).

M.B. lived at home until the age of 105 and then entered a nursing home. According to her family, it was still possible to have meaningful conversations with her until the age of 110. According to the nursing home, meaningful exchanges took place until her death even if she had good days and bad days. M.B. was a rebel, according to the nursing home staff (personal communication). They give the following example. M.B. was always refusing a hearing aid for the reason that, according to her, she could hear the nurses perfectly. For her 113th birthday the nursing home prepared a big public party without asking her permission. Consequently she refused to come to the party. For the birthdays following this one, the staff of the nursing home asked her opinion and organized intimate parties. After her 115th birthday, she worried about how she could answer the emails received for her birthday.

In summary, these seven supercentenarians lived on average 116.9 years, of which 108.1 were spent in the community, 92.5 % of their total life expectancy, with 8.8 years spent in a retirement community or nursing home (7.5 % of their life). Out of seven, only one was suspected to be demented before death[2] and five remained mentally alert until their death, according to their informants, if we exclude the last weeks of their life.

In this paper we have examined the state of knowledge on longevity and cognition and particularly the cognitive status of supercentenarians, those having reached at least the age of 110. We established that our current knowledge about the cognitive status of the oldest old is based on extrapolation from mainly younger populations. We also addressed the question of what we mean by good cognitive function at extreme ages, and chose the presence of meaningful conversation as an indicator of good cognitive function for supercentenarians. We then reported the cases of seven persons who had recently reached or surpassed the age of 115, six women and one man whose ages had been carefully validated. These case studies show that, if we exclude the final days or weeks of life, dementia is not inevitable at extreme ages. Of course, we cannot say that our cases were not demented at all. Obviously J.C. and S.K. had memory problems and had showed a steady decline in the last years of their life compared to how they were a few years before. However, they remained capable of meaningful conversation until the last year of their life.

If we consider that the capacity to have a meaningful conversation indicates the absence of significant cognitive decline, our observations allow us to dismiss any kind of exponential trajectory to summarize the relationship between age and cognitive decline among the oldest old. In fact, using this criterion of meaningful conversation, the cognitive status of the supercentenarians appears to be excellent, even better than that of the centenarians described above with

---

[2] This is the case of M.L.M, whose dementia seemed to appear and develop between the ages of 112 and 116. According to a nurse (M.D.) who knew M.L.M. from the time of her admission to the nursing home, M.L.M. was in very good health and able to have intelligent and meaningful conversation when she entered the nursing home at the age of 107. The first episodes of confusion took place when she was 112 years old and seemed to be associated with sensory problems (she had become almost deaf and totally lost the vision in one eye). At the age of 113, she was often resistive and argumentative, especially related to care tasks. She was very religious and spent a lot of time praying. She was often heard to ask God why he had not come to get her. She was alternating in her last years between sleep and periods of lucidity, during which she would most often pray. She would also talk sometimes about fishing and her recipe for longevity "attending church and never letting a man dominate your life." According to M.D., M.L.M. deteriorated rapidly the year before she died (B. Desjardins, personal communication).

traditional screening instruments, such as the SPMSE or the MMSE, if it is possible to establish an equivalence between three or more errors to the SPMSE and being unable to have a meaningful conversation. This perhaps gives more support to a quadratic trajectory than a logistic one. However, it is probable that supercentenarians, as well as centenarians, have been in part selected for their higher cognitive abilities through the mortality process (see Maier et al. this volume), changing the cognitive composition of the population with ageing and such changes may explain logistic and even quadratic trajectories. Thus, although we still cannot differentiate *the exact for of* the relationship between cognitive decline and age, we have provided some evidence that dementia at advanced ages is not a certainty.

Acknowledgments

We acknowledge Bertrand Desjardins, Peter Laslett, Margery Silver, and John Wilmoth who provided the information used in this paper and Jacki Smith who commented on the notion of meaningful conversation.

References

Allard M (1991) A la recherche du secret des centenaires. Le Cherche Midi Editeur, Paris.

Allard M, Robine JM (2000) Les centenaires français. Etude de la Fondation IPSEN, 1990–2000. Serdi Edition, Paris.

Andersen-Ranberg K, Vasegaard L, Jeune B (2001) Dementia is not inevitable: a population based study of Danish centenarians. J Gerontol: Psychosoc Sci 56B (3): P152–159.

Beregi E, Klinger A (1989) Health and living conditions of centenarians in Hungary. Int Psychogeriat 1: 195–200.

Blansjaar BA, Thomassen R, van Schaik HW (2000) Prevalence of dementia in centenarians. Int J Geriat Psychiat 15: 219–225.

DesJardins B (1999) Did Marie Louise Meilleur become the oldest person in the world. In: Jeune B, Vaupel JW (eds) Validation of exceptional longevity. Odense Monographs on Population Aging 6, Odense University Press, Odense, 189–194.

Dewey ME, Copeland JRM (2001) Dementia in centenarians. Int J Geriat Psychiat 16: 538–539.

Fondation IPSEN (1991) 100 tableaux pour 100 ans. A la recherche du secret des centenaires, Document n° 1, Fondation Ipsen, Paris.

Freedman VA, Aykan H, Martin LG (2001) Aggregate changes in severe cognitive impairment among older Americans: 1993 and 1998. J GerontolSoc Sci 56B (5): S100–S111.

Hagberg B, Bauer Alfredson B, Poon LW, Homma A (2001) Cognitive functioning in centenarians: a coordinated analysis of results from three countries. J Gerontol Psychosoc Sci 56B (3): P141–151.

Jorm AF, Korten AE, Henderson AS (1987) The prevalence of dementia: a quantitative integration of the literature. Acta Psychiatr Scand 76: 465–79

Louhija J (1994) Finnish centenarians: A clinical epidemiological study. Helsinki, Finland: Yliopistopaino.

Pfeiffer EA (1975) Short Portable Mental Status Questionnaire for the assessment of organic brain deficit in elderly patients. J. Am Geriatr Soc 23: 440.

Preston GAN (1986) Dementia in elderly adults: prevalence and institutionalisation. J Gerontol 41: 261–267

Ritchie K (1995) Mental status examination of an exceptional case of longevity J.C. aged 118 years. Brit J Psychiatr 166: 229–235.

Ritchie K, Kildea D (1995) Is senile dementia 'age related' or 'ageing related'? Evidence from meta-analysis of dementia prevalence in oldest old. Lancet 346: 931–934.

Ritchie K, Kildea D, Robine J-M (1992) The relationship between age and the prevalence of senile dementia: a meta-analysis of recent data. Int J Epidemiol 21: 763–769.

Robine JM, Allard M (1998) The oldest human. Science 279: 1834–1835.

Robine JM, Allard M (1999) Jeanne Calment : validation of the duration of her life. In: Jeune B, Vaupel JW (Eds) Validation of exceptional longevity. Odense Monographs on Population Aging 6, Odense University Press, Odense, pp. 145–172.

Robine JM, Vaupel JW (2001) Supercentenarians, slower ageing individuals or senile elderly? Exp Gerontol L 36 (4–6): 915–930.

Robine JM, Vaupel JW (2002) Emergence of supercentenarians in low mortality countries. North American Actuarial J, in press

Robine JM, Romieu I, Michel JP (2002) Trends in health expectancies. In: Robine JM, Jagger C, Crimmins et al. (eds) Determining health expectancies. Wiley, Chichester, in press

Rodgers Mayer E (Phoebe Ministries, 1997).

Silver MH, Jilinskaia E, Perls TT (2001) Cognitive functional status of age-confirmed centenarians in a population-based study. J Gerontol Psychosoc Sci 56B (3): P134–140.

Thatcher AR (1999 b). The long-term pattern of adult mortality and the highest attained age. J R Stat Soc 162: 43.

Vaupel JW, Jeune B (1995) The emergence and proliferation of centenarians. In: Jeune B, Vaupel JW (eds) Exceptional longevity: from prehistory to the present. Odense Monographs on Population Aging 2, Odense University Press, Odense, pp. 109–116.

Vaupel JW, Carey JR, Christensen K, Johnson TE, Yashin Al, Holm NV, Iachine IA, Kannisto V, Khazaeli AA, Liedo P, Longo VD, Yi Zeng, Manton KG, Curtsinger JW (1998). Biodemographic trajectories of longevity. Science 280: 855–860.

Wilmoth JR, Skytthe A, Friou D, Jeune B (1996) The oldest man ever? A case study of exceptional longevity. Gerontologist 36 (6): 783–788.

IQ at Age 11 and Longevity: Results from a Follow-Up of the Scottish Mental Survey 1932

I. J. Deary[1], *L. J. Whalley*[2] and *J. M. Starr*[3]

Summary

Childhood social factors – such as education, occupational status and relative social deprivation – are known to affect longevity. Mental ability differences in childhood are related to these social factors. However, there are few studies of the association between mental ability in childhood and survival. Here we examine the association between IQ at age 11 and survival to age 76 in a follow-up study of the Scottish Mental Survey of 1932 (SMS 1932). In the SMS 1932 all children born in 1921 and attending school in Scotland on June 1, 1932 were given the same valid mental ability test (an IQ-type test) under the same conditions. We chose the 2792 children from schools in the Aberdeen area of Scotland as our target population. We searched public and health records in Scotland, England and Wales to discover whether they had died or were still alive on January 1, 1997. Copies of death certificates were obtained. Deaths certified as due to cancer were noted. The association between childhood IQ and survival was studied using Cox proportional hazards regression (Whalley and Deary 2001). People with higher childhood IQ scores tended to live longer. The association differed between the sexes. The association in women was maintained across the life span. In men, the association was reversed during World War II: those with a higher IQ had a higher risk of dying during that period. Controlling for overcrowding in the person's school area did not account for the association between IQ and survival. In the present report we examine for the first time the odds ratios of survival for IQ groups (divided into quartiles) for men and women. We find evidence of a deleterious effect of low IQ and a protective effect of belonging to the highest IQ group. The association between childhood IQ and risk of death from cancer is examined. Dying from cancer, and more specifically stomach and lung cancers, is associated with lower childhood IQ scores.

---

[1] Department of Psychology, University of Edinburgh, 7 George Square, Edinburgh EH8 9JZ, Scotland, UK
[2] Department of Mental Health, University of Aberdeen, Clinical Research Centre, Cornhill Hospital, Aberdeen AB24 2ZD, Scotland, UK
[3] Department of Geriatric Medicine, Royal Victoria Hospital, Craigleith Road, Edinburgh EH4 2DN, Scotland, UK

Finch et al. (Eds.)
Brain and Longevity
© Springer-Verlag Berlin Heidelberg 2003

Introduction

The present report concerns the association between childhood IQ and longevity. It reports several new findings from our research programme which follows up the Scottish Mental Survey 1932 (Deary et al. 2000). Specifically, we report here supplementary analyses to our previous study of IQ and survival (Whalley and Deary 2001), and we examine the association between IQ in childhood and death from cancer.

Education, socio-economic status and mental ability are moderately strongly correlated (Jencks et al. 1979; Scullin et al. 2000). Higher mental ability is associated with more education and relatively advantageous socioeconomic status (Neisser et al. 1996). However, only for education and socio-economic status do many data exist with respect to their influence on human morbidity and mortality. People who live in relatively deprived social conditions have higher rates of illnesses – such as cardiovascular diseases and cancers – and tend to die younger (Black 1980; Duijkers et al. 1989; Eames et al. 1993; Fox et al. 1985; McLoone and Boddy 1994). Childhood social circumstances show significant associations with several major illnesses in adulthood, including coronary heart disease, stroke, lung cancer, stomach cancer, and respiratory disease (Davey Smith et al. 1998 a; Joseph and Kramer 1996). The age at which people leave full-time education also relates to death from cancer and cardiovascular disease and to deaths that are not from these causes (Davey Smith et al. 1998 b). In the Nun Study, those sisters who were educated to bachelor degree level or higher lived, on average, about seven years longer than those whose education was to college, high school or grade school level (Snowdon et al. 1989). The odds ratio of the nuns with degrees surviving and being independent of nursing services in old age was over 2.5 when compared with all less-educated nuns.

There are relatively few established associations between personal traits and human morbidity and mortality. An exception is the small influence that individual differences in hostility have upon the risk of cardiovascular disease (Whiteman et al. 2000). Studies of the far-from-representative "Terman Life Cycle of Children with High Ability" sample (N = 1258) found that the personality traits of conscientiousness, lack of cheerfulness and permanence of mood (for men only in this latter case) were associated with living longer (Schwartz et al. 1995).

Among older people, cognitive status and amount of cognitive decline within old age may be a predictor of mortality (Deeg et al. 1990; Korten et al. 1999). Mental ability was predictive of survival in a study of Vietnam veterans after discharge, though they were still relatively young when the study was conducted (O'Toole and Stankov 1992).

Mental ability from young adulthood was predictive of survival within old age in the Nun Study (Snowdon et al. 1999). The "idea density" measure from nuns' handwritten autobiographies in early life (in the 1930 s and 1940 s) was related to likelihood of survival in the surveillance period between 1991 and

1998, during which 58 of the 180 subjects died. There was a relative risk of death of about 1.5 with each unit decrease in idea density. The relationship was not altered by controlling for education, but disappeared after controlling for Mini-Mental State Examination score in late life. The effect whereby idea density was linked to survival within old age was limited to the bottom quartile of ability. This lowest ability group had the lowest survival rates. The upper three quartiles had similar survival patterns. Applying their findings to a hypothetical group of 75-year-olds, Snowdon et al. (1999) calculated that, whereas only 17 % of 75-year-olds with low idea density survived to age 90, 43 % of those with high idea density would survive. Because the nuns in their sample had very similar adult environments and lifestyles, they argued that the association between idea density and survival within old age was caused by "linguistic and cognitive abilities of the participants in early life," and not "lifestyle and environmental risk factors present during mid and late adult life" (p. 112).

Research with The Scottish Mental Survey 1932

The Scottish Mental Survey of 1932 (SMS 1932; Scottish Council for Research in Education [SCRE] 1933) administered a group test of mental ability (a version of the Moray House Test No. 12) to all children attending school in Scotland on June 1, 1932 and born in 1921 (N = 87,498). Very few schools failed to take part. Those children who were absent owing to illness were not tested. Therefore, Scotland has valid IQ data for almost the entire birth cohort of 1921. The test had a variety of types of item (see Deary et al. 2000). The maximum possible score on the test was 76. The test's time limit was 45 minutes. Scores on this Moray House Test correlated almost 0.8 with the individually administered Stanford-Binet test in a large, near-representative sample of the SMS 1932 (N = 1,000).

The Scottish Council for Research in Education retained the SMS 1932 data and the present authors have employed them to examine the effects of cognitive ability in early life on health in later life. To date we have reported that:
- mental ability differences are relatively stable from age 11 to age 77 (Deary et al. 2000)
- mental ability at age 11 is significantly associated with the risk of senile but not presenile dementia in later life (Whalley et al. 2000)
- mental ability at age 11 is significantly related to self-rated disability in old age (Starr et al. 2000).

In addition, using the SMS 1932 data, we showed that mental ability test scores at age 11 were significantly related to survival during the period from June 1, 1932 to January 1, 1997, i.e., from age 11 up to age 76 years (Whalley and Deary 2001). This conclusion was based on a Cox regression analysis of the 2230 persons traced (to "dead", "alive" or "moved away") from the 2792 people who took the SMS 1932 test in the Aberdeen area of Scotland. The association was not substantially altered by controlling for overcrowding in the school's catchment area. The effect across the life span was clearer in women, because men who died during World War II had a relatively high mean IQ score. For example, women with a one standard deviation disadvantage in IQ score were, on average, only 71 % as likely to be alive at age 76 than those with the higher IQ (95 % confidence interval = 64 % to 78 %).

The present report extends the above study (Whalley and Deary 2001) of the relation between mental ability in early life and survival across the human life span to old age. It contains the following novel analyses. First, we present survival data for men and women divided into four quartiles of IQ score at age 11 years. This is to test whether, as found by Snowdon et al. (1999), the relation between early life ability and survival is largely a result of lower survival of people in the lowest quartile of IQ scores. These data are analysed as odds ratios. Second, we present new data on the association between IQ at age 11 and death from cancer in general. Third, we present new data on the association between IQ at age 11 and death from specific cancers, especially lung cancer. These analyses are a partial attempt to examine whether early life mental ability differences have the same relation to specific causes of death as do socioeconomic conditions in childhood (Davey Smith et al. 1998 a).

Sample and analyses

The present analyses of childhood IQ and health are extensions of the analyses that appeared in Whalley and Deary (2001). The target population is the 2792 people from Aberdeen schools who took part in the Scottish Mental Survey of 1932. The working sample is the 79.9 % of those people whose status was traced at January 1, 1997 (total N = 2230). Their status allocations on that date were "dead", "alive" or "moved away" (with date of moving). Since the publication by Whalley and Deary (2001) we have incorporated some small amendments to the database as new information was received about status of subjects on 1/1/97. For the analyses of all cause mortality (requiring an actual year of death) there were full data for 2171 subjects. For the analyses of cancer deaths there were between 2181 and 2185 subjects with relevant data. Details of statistical analyses are described with the results. Analyses were performed on a PC running SPSS 10.1, except for odds ratios and their 95 % confidence intervals, which were calculated from the formulae provided by Bland and Altman (2000).

Results

IQ at Age 11 and Death by 1/1/97

Survival curves to 1/1/97 for the four quartiles based upon IQ differences measured at age 11 years on 1/6/32 are shown separately for women and men in Figures 1 a und 1 b, respectively.

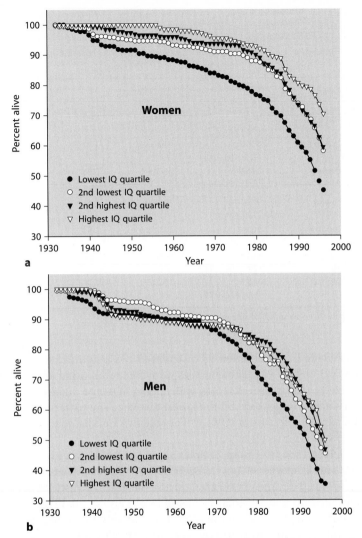

Fig. 1. Percentage of surviving subjects from the Scottish Mental Survey of 1932 at ages between 12 and 76 years for: women in the four IQ score quartiles (Fig. 1 a) and men in the four IQ score quartiles (Fig. 1 b). Mental ability test scores were obtained at age 11 years

For women, as shown previously (Whalley and Deary 2001), there is an early and sustained difference in survival to 1/1/97 between the highest and lowest quartiles of IQ as measured at age 11 years on 1/6/32. The two middle quartiles fall at intermediate survival levels throughout the period of the life span examined here, with little difference between them, especially in old age. The numbers of women alive and dead at 1/1/97 within the four IQ quartiles are shown in Table 1 (top). Contingency table analysis for the proportions of

Table 1. Odds ratios ($\pm$ 95 % confidence intervals) for death by 1/1/97 and IQ at age 11. IQs were grouped as quartiles and the top three quartiles were compared with the lowest IQ quartile

	IQ quartile	Mean IQ (SD; range[a])	N dead/alive at 1/1/97	Odds ratio	Odds ratio's 95 % CI
Women	Lowest	79.9 (8.2; 58–90)	150/123	1.0	
	2nd lowest	96.7 (3.3; 91–102)	112/155	1.69	1.20 to 2.37
	2nd highest	106.3 (2.5; 102–111)	110/160	1.77	1.26 to 2.50
	Highest	116.9 (5.0; 111–134)	66/156	2.88	1.98 to 4.19
Men	Lowest	79.3 (7.8; 60–91)	181/99	1.0	
	2nd lowest	96.8 (3.0; 91–102)	153/128	1.52	1.08 to 2.14
	2nd highest	106.3 (2.6; 102–111)	148/129	1.59	1.13 to 2.23
	Highest	118.3 (5.9; 111–139)	151/150	1.81	1.29 to 2.52

[a] IQ ranges have been rounded to integers

women surviving in the different IQ quartiles shows a significant difference (χ^2 = 32.5, d.f. = 3, p < 0.001). The quartiles were compared using analysis of odds ratios (Table 1). The three quartiles with higher IQs had significantly greater likelihoods of surviving than did the lowest quartile. The pattern of odds ratios suggests a similar effect from IQ 91 to 111 (the two middle quartiles) and a yet greater effect at high levels of IQ.

Among men there is a more complex association between survival to 1/1/97 and IQ measured at age 11 on 1/6/32 (Fig. 1 b). The two highest IQ quartile groups show steep declines in survival during the years of World War II. Thereafter, they catch up and eventually emerge in old age as the highest-surviving groups. After about 1970, when the subjects are about to turn 50, the lowest IQ quartile group has the lowest percentage survival. The numbers of men alive and dead at 1/1/97 within the four IQ quartiles are shown in Table 1 (bottom). Contingency table analysis for the proportions of men surviving in the different IQ quartiles shows a significant difference (χ^2 = 13.6, d.f. = 3, p = 0.004). The quartiles were compared using analysis of odds ratios (Table 1). The lowest IQ quartile was used as the reference group. The three quartiles with higher IQs had significantly greater likelihoods of surviving to 1/1/97 than did the lowest IQ quartile. The pattern of odds ratios suggests a relatively similar effect from IQ 91 to 139 (the two middle quartiles and the upper quartile). However, the relatively greater specific impact of World War II on the higher two IQ quartiles may mask a similar effect to that found among women, whereby the highest IQ quartile survived more than the middle two quartiles.

IQ at Age 11 and Death by Cancer by 1/1/97

The next analysis on these data was based on a death certificate entry of any type of cancer as a cause of death. The numbers of Aberdeen City people who sat the Scottish Mental Survey test in June 1932 and who had or had not died of a cancer death by 1/1/97 were examined. Among women, those (N = 159) dying of cancer by 1/1/97 had a significantly lower IQ (mean = 96.0, standard deviation = 14.1) compared with those (N = 873) who did not (mean IQ = 99.7, standard deviation = 14.4; t = 2.98, d.f. = 1030, p = 0.003). Among men, those (N = 172) dying of cancer by 1/1/97 had a significantly lower IQ (mean = 97.2, standard deviation = 16.4) compared with those (N = 981) who did not (mean IQ = 101.0, standard deviation = 15.1; p = 0.003). The numbers of those dying of cancer are listed by quartile of IQ score obtained at age 11, separately for women and men, in Table 2. Among women a contingency table analysis suggests an increasing number of deaths from cancer in the lower IQ groups (χ^2 = 10.9, d.f. = 3, p = 0.01). A similar difference between proportions of cancer deaths in the different IQ quartiles is found among men (χ^2 = 8.9, d.f. = 3, p = 0.03).

An analysis of odds ratios was carried out on the numbers of cancer deaths in the different IQ quartiles (Table 2). The lowest IQ quartile was used as the reference group. The direction of the odds ratio is such as to indicate surviving and not dying from cancer. Thus, a higher odds ratio is better. Among women, the middle two quartiles had an odds ratio of about 1.5, though only the second lowest quartile achieved the conventional level of statistical significance (p < 0.05; i.e., the 95 % confidence interval did not cross 1.0). The female quartile with the highest IQ had an odds ratio of 2.28 and these people were thus less than half as likely to die of cancer as those in the lowest IQ quartile. Among men, the highest two quartiles were significantly less likely to die of cancer in the surveillance period with similar odds ratios of about 1.8.

Table 2. Odds ratios (± 95 % confidence intervals) for death by cancer by 1/1/97 and IQ at age 11. IQs were grouped as quartiles and the top three quartiles were compared with the lowest IQ quartile.

	IQ quartile	N for all cancer deaths/all others by 1/1/97	Odds ratio for all cancer deaths/ all others by 1/1/97	Odds ratio's 95 % CI	N lung cancer deaths by 1/1/97
Women	Lowest	57/216	1.0		15
	2nd lowest	38/229	1.59	1.01 to 2.50	5
	2nd highest	41/229	1.47	0.95 to 2.29	9
	Highest	23/199	2.28	1.36 to 3.84	5
Men	Lowest	57/228	1.0		25
	2nd lowest	43/240	1.40	0.90 to 2.16	15
	2nd highest	34/243	1.79	1.13 to 2.83	16
	Highest	38/269	1.77	1.32 to 2.77	8

Cox proportional hazards analysis also suggested that the IQ score at age 11 was associated with death by cancer: among women, p < 0.001, regression coefficient = –0.022 (standard error = 0.005), change in relative rates for each IQ point = 0.978 (95 % confidence interval = 0.968 to 0.988); and among men, p = 0.001, regression coefficient = – 0.016 (standard error = 0.005), change in relative rates for each IQ point = 0.984 (95 % confidence interval = 0.974 to 0.994). Thus, a one standard deviation (15 points) disadvantage entails an approximately 40 % increase in chance of death by cancer among women and a 27 % increase among men.

IQ at Age 11 and Death by Specific Cancers and Lung Cancer by 1/1/97

Instances of specific cancers were noted from death certificates. Those cancers with total occurrences equal to or greater than 12 cases, as noted on death certificates, were used for further analysis. This included a category where "cancer" was noted without further specification. The mean childhood IQ (standard error) of each of these cancer groups is shown in Figure 2. One-way analysis of variance was used to compare the mean IQ of each cancer group with the mean IQ of those people who did not die of cancer by 1/1/97. Overall, those who had died of cancer by 1/1/97 had lower IQs (F = 3.15, d.f. = 7,2184, p = 0.003). Planned comparisons among groups showed that the groups with stomach, lung and unspecified cancer had lower mean IQs than the group who did not die of cancer (see Fig. 2).

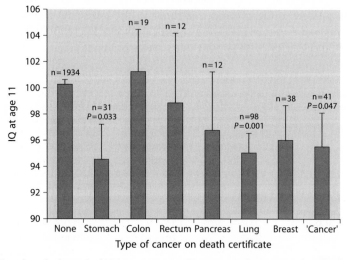

Fig. 2. Mean (standard error) of IQ in groups according to type of cancer noted on death certificate, compared with all other traced (alive and dead) members of the sample. P values are the result of planned (LSD) comparisons between the specific cancer mortality group and the members (surviving and deceased) of the sample who did not die of cancer

The final analyses concerned those people who died of lung cancer by 1/1/ 97. The numbers of men and women who died of lung cancer by 1/1/97 for each IQ quartile are shown in Table 2. Contingency table analyses showed that more men in the lower IQ groups died of lung cancer (χ^2 = 10.8, d.f. = 3, p = 0.01). There was no significant effect among women (χ^2 = 6.6, d.f. = 3, p = 0.09).

Comment

The present results extend our previous findings of an association between mental ability differences in early life and differences in longevity (Whalley and Deary 2001). There are cohort-specific effects here that limit the generalisability of the results. Principal among these is the association between death in active service in World War II and relatively high IQ. This, though, serves to demonstrate that any association between mental ability in early life and survival is not immutable. Among women, where a war-specific effect was absent, there was a suggestion that the lowest and highest IQ quartiles had contrasting survival odds ratios compared with the middle two quartiles, which were similar. This finding differs from the Snowdon et al. (1999) Nun Study's finding of an effect of early life ability on longevity that was limited to the lowest quartile. The comparability of the two studies is limited, however. Snowdon and colleagues limited the surveillance epoch to a period of about a decade within old age and their sample of nuns was highly selected, contrasting with the near-normal population sample examined here.

The present data also add new findings to the study of childhood factors in relation to death from cancers. Davey Smith and colleagues (1998 b) found that stomach and lung cancer deaths among men aged 35–64 years in the West of Scotland were related to a father's occupational group, i.e., to the subjects' childhood socio-economic status. The association between father's occupational grouping and stomach cancer, but not for lung cancer, remained significant when the subject's own occupational status in adult life was controlled. They concluded that mortality from stomach, but not lung, cancer was in part influenced by childhood factors, for example the likehood of infection by *H. pylori*, and not merely by a continuity of social disadvantage from childhood to adult life. In the same sample, the same research team found that the age at which people left full-time education was related to the likelihood of dying from cancer (Davey Smith et al. 1998 b). Future research must inquire after the "active ingredient" among the cognitive and socio-economic status variables that is responsible for this association.

Elsewhere we have speculated on some of the mechanisms that might account for the association between childhood IQ and longevity (Whalley and Deary 2001). Two of the hypothesised mechanisms were influences of childhood IQ on adult lifestyle. On the one hand, differences in childhood mental ability might be associated with lifestyle choices such as smoking, drinking, diet, and dangerous activities. The latter suggestion accords with the finding that the trait of conscientiousness is associated with longer life (Schwartz et al. 1995). On the other hand, higher childhood IQ might afford entry to work and other environments that are generally safer. While these part-explanations seem reasonable, even obvious, there are other suggestions for the association, along the lines of childhood IQ acting as a marker for the integrity of the organism, even as early as 11 years. The evidence that "programming" in the foetus might affect adult illnesses, and the association between birth weight and length and later IQ in the SMS 1932 subjects (Shenkin et al. 2001), are supportive of this type of suggestion. Similarly, Snowdon et al. (1989), when they reported the association between linguistic ability in early life and survival within old age, suggested that

> "Low linguistic ability in early life may reflect suboptimal neurological and cognitive development that might increase susceptibility to aging-related declines and disease processes late in life" (p. 112).

Thus childhood IQ might have direct effects on health and longevity as well as effects that are mediated via adult lifestyle and environments. In amassing these possible paths between childhood IQ and longevity (Fig. 3), we were struck by the similarity with the model of Poon et al. (1997), whose Figure 3 came to our notice after our own was prepared. In a similar fashion to our proposal, Poon et al. (1997) suggest that individual differences in intelligence may act as antecedent, mediating, and outcome variables with respect to health, and that intelligence may be a cause as well as a consequence of health-related environments. It is the construction and rigorous testing of such sophisticated models that will be important in future research.

Our current research with the Scottish Mental Survey 1932 data includes plans to examine associations between childhood IQ and all-cause mortality

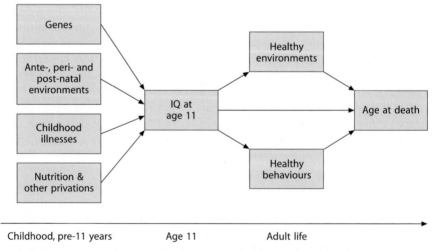

Fig. 3. Possible paths for the association between childhood mental ability and mortality: mental ability may act as a dependent, mediating and/or independent variable

and specific causes of mortality for the whole birth cohort. This work will improve the generalisability of the present results beyond the geographic area we have studied here. However, these larger-scale analyses will still contain cohort-specific effects.

Acknowledgements

The research reported here was supported by grants to the authors from Henry Smith's Charity (LJW), the Biotechnology and Biological Sciences Research Council (IJD, LJW and JMS), and the Scottish Executive Health Department Chief Scientist's Office (IJD, LJW and JMS). We thank David Hunter, Duncan Leitch, Elizabeth Whalley, Patricia Whalley, and Margaret Rush for assistance with the gathering and compiling of data. We thank Valerie Wilson and Graham Thorpe from the Scottish Council for Research in Education for allowing access to the Scottish Mental Survey 1932 data. We thank Rebecca Fuhrer for suggesting the odds ratio analyses of IQ and mortality.

References

Black D (1980) Inequalities in health: Report of a working group chaired by Sir Douglas Black. Department of Health and Social Security. London

Bland JM, Altman DG (2000) The odds ratio. Brit Med J 320: 1468

Davey Smith G, Hart C, Blane D, Hole D (1998 a) Adverse socioeconomic conditions in childhood and cause specific adult mortality: prospective observational study. Brit Med J 316: 1631–1635

Davey Smith G, Hart C, Hole D, MacKinnon P, Gillis C, Watt G, Blane D, Hawthorne V (1998 b) Education and occupational social class: which is the more important indicator of mortality risk? J Epidemiol Commun Health 52: 153–160

Deary IJ, Whalley LJ, Lemmon H, Crawford JR, Starr JM (2000) The stability of individual differences in mental ability from childhood to old age: follow-up of the 1932 Scottish Mental Survey. Intelligence 28: 49–55

Deeg DJH, Hofman A, Zonneveld J van (1990) The association between change in cognitive function and longevity in Dutch elderly. Am J Epidemiol 132: 973–982

Duijkers TJ, Kromhout D, Spruit IP, Doornbos G (1989) Inter-mediating risk factors in the relation between socioeconomic status and 25-year mortality (the Zutphen study). Intl J Epidemiol 18: 658–662

Eames M, Ben-Shlomo Y, Marmot MG (1993) Social deprivation and premature mortality: regional comparison across England. Brit Med J 307: 1097–1102

Fox AJ, Goldblatt PO, Jones DR (1985) Social class mortality differentials: artefact, selection or life circumstances? J Epidemiol Commun Health 39: 1–18

Jencks C, Bartlett S, Corcoran M, Crouse J, Eaglesfield D, Jackson G, McClelland K, Mueser P, Olneck M, Schwartz J, Ward S, Williams J (1979) Who gets ahead? The determinants of economic success in America. Basic Books, New York

Joseph KS, Kramer MS (1996) Review of the evidence on fetal and early childhood antecedents of adult chronic disease. Epidemiol Rev 18: 158–174

Korten AE, Jorm AF, Jiao Z, Letenneur L, Jacomb PA, Henderson AS, Christensen H, Rogers B (1999) Health, cognitive and psychosocial factors as predictors of mortality in an elderly community sample. J Epidemiol Commun Health 53: 83–88

McLoone P, Boddy FA (1994) Deprivation and mortality in Scotland, 1981 and 1991. Brit Med J 309: 1465–1470

Neisser U, Boodoo G, Bouchard TJ, Boykin AW, Brody N, Ceci SJ, Halpern DF, Loehlin JC, Perloff R, Sternberg RJ, Urbina S (1996) Intelligence: knowns and unknowns. Am Psychol 51: 77–101

O'Toole BI, Stankov L (1992) Ultimate validity of psychological tests. Personality Individual Differences 13: 699–716

Poon LW, Johnson MA, Martin P (1997) Looking into the crystal ball: will we ever be able to accurately predict individual differences in longevity. In: Robine J-M, Vaupel JW, Jeune B, Allard M (eds) Longevity: to the limits and beyond. New York, Springer, pp. 113–119

Schwartz JE, Friedman HS, Tucker JS, Tomlinson-Keasey C, Wingard DL, Criqui MH (1995) Sociodemographic and psychosocial factors in childhood as predictors of adult mortality? Am J Publ Health 85: 1237–1245

Scottish Council for Research in Education (1933) The intelligence of Scottish children: a national survey of an age-group. University of London Press, London

Scullin MH, Peters E, Williams WM, Ceci SJ (2000) The role of IQ and education in predicting later labor market outcomes. Psychol, Publ Policy Law 6: 63–89

Shenkin SD, Starr JM, Pattie A, Rush MA, Whalley LJ, Deary IJ (2001) Birth weight and cognitive function at age 11 years: The Scottish Mental Survey 1932. Arch of Dis Childhood 85: 189–197

Snowdon DA, Ostwald SK, Kane RL (1989) Education, survival, and independence in elderly Catholic sisters, 1936–1988. Am J Epidemiol 130: 999–1012

Snowdon DA, Greiner LH, Kemper SJ, Nanayakkara N, Mortimer JA (1999) Linguistic ability in early life and longevity: findings from the Nun Study. In: Robine J-M, Forette B, Franceschi C, Allard M (eds) The paradoxes of longevity. New York, Springer, pp. 103–113

Starr JM, Deary IJ, Lemmon H, Whalley LJ (2000) Mental ability age 11 years and health status age 77 years. Age Ageing 29: 523–528

Whalley LJ, Deary IJ (2001) Longitudinal cohort study of childhood IQ and survival up to age 76. Brit Med J 322: 1–5

Whalley LJ, Starr JM, Athawes R, Hunter D, Pattie A, Deary IJ (2000) Childhood mental ability and dementia. Neurology 55: 1455-1459

Whiteman MC, Deary IJ, Fowkes FGR (2000) Personality and health: cardiovascular disease. In: Hampson S (ed) Advances in personality psychology Vol 1. Psychology Press, London, pp. 157–198

Paths to Longevity in the Highly Intelligent Terman Cohort

H. S. Friedman and Ch.N. Markey

Summary

Although highly intelligent people may have certain advantages in maintaining health, there are no simple or strong relationships between intelligence and longevity. This chapter analyses the risks to longevity among 1528 highly intelligent children who were first studied by Lewis Terman in 1922 when they were about 10 years old. All the children had IQs of at least 135 and were good students. Data assessing their substance use, mental health, life stress, social relations, and personality have been collected and refined. Importantly, we have collected death certificates. Findings suggest that although this cohort lives longer than average, these intelligent people faced many of the challenges and threats to health faced by ordinary people. Health-related behaviors (substance use), psychological adjustment, personality, and social relationships are all important predictors of longevity. We conclude that while intelligent people may have certain advantages in maintaining their health, they are not invincible to the key behavioral and psychosocial influences that interact with biology to determine mortality risk. Going beyond biology, the broader patterns of individual life paths need to be taken into account in understanding longevity and in designing health-relevant interventions.

> "We should take care not to make the intellect our God; it has, of course, powerful muscles, but no personality." – *Albert Einstein*
> ("Religion and Science," New York Times Magazine, 9 November, 1930)

Popular stereotypes of highly intelligent people contrast them with athletes, tough guys and manual laborers. The highly intelligent may be labeled as frail, weak, and "nerdy" as compared to their muscular, robust counterparts. Despite such clichés, there is little empirical research that suggests that intelligent people are frail or experience poor health. In fact, research suggests that intelligence is inversely related to morbidity and mortality; bright people live longer. The strength of the relationship between health and intelligence is not decisively strong, however. It turns out that intelligence may serve as a marker for other health factors, and although it potentially provides a number of health advantages, these advantages are often outweighed by other factors. There is a complex network of moderating factors that need consideration.

Finch et al. (Eds.)
Brain and Longevity
© Springer-Verlag Berlin Heidelberg 2003

This issue is not a new one. In 1922, Lewis Terman, a psychologist at Stanford University, set out to study the life-course of highly intelligent individuals (Terman 1925). Terman did not believe the stereotype of the weak, ineffective genius who was predestined to be a geek or nerd. On the contrary, influenced by Charles Darwin, Terman was looking to see if the most intelligent among us could become the strong, vigorous leaders needed to save civilization. To this end, Terman did something quite unusual for his time. He launched a comprehensive, longitudinal study of gifted children.

Longitudinal data make it clear that health is not a static quality; health takes a dynamic course that is a result of developmental processes influenced by biological, behavioral, and psychosocial factors. Further, there is a bi-directional nature of potential relations between intelligence and health that must be considered. This chapter employs Terman's life-span data set to explore highly intelligent individuals' development, patterns of health behaviors, psychological make-up, and social experiences, in relation to their longevity.

The Terman Data

The Terman Life Cycle Study began with 1528 elementary school children in an effort to describe the life course of gifted individuals (Terman and Oden 1947). This data set is a rich source of information about individuals' paths through life, their health, and longevity. Continued until the present, it is the longest comprehensive study of a large cohort ever conducted, and the only such major study with rich data collected regularly throughout the life span (from childhood until death). Together with our colleagues (especially Kathleen Clark, Michael Criqui, Leslie Martin, Joseph Schwartz, Carol Tomlinson-Keasey, and Joan Tucker), we have made major efforts to follow up on and improve the dataset. Data have been collected and refined on the subjects' health behaviors, social relations, personalities, careers, families, mental health, and life stress; importantly, we have collected death certificates (Friedman et al. 1995 b).

This sample is relatively homogeneous on dimensions of intelligence and social class. All participants were tested as having an IQ of 135 or greater before beginning participation in the study, and participants predominantly maintained productive, middle-class lives throughout adulthood. The homogeneous nature of this sample does not lend itself to be easily generalized to the U.S. population as a whole. However, these characteristics of this sample insure that participants were capable of understanding medical advice and had access to health care. Overall, there is an extremely low attrition rate of 6 % for this sample, leaving us very complete information about the Terman sample. These data provide us with a unique window into the lives of highly intelligent people born almost a century ago.

Biological Influences on Paths to Longevity

From a biological viewpoint, it makes sense to assume that intelligent people will be healthier and live longer. For example, IQ has been posited as an indirect measure of both bodily insults and system integrity (Whalley and Deary 2001). Highly intelligent, "cognitively healthy" individuals should have superior physical health. First, individuals' life courses are determined initially by biological growth and early experiences. Genetic predispositions and prenatal development influence the growth of both brains and bodies. Healthy early developmental experiences combined with robust genes set the stage for both high-functioning brains and long-living bodies.

Second, intelligence reflects efficient information processing and nervous system activity, both of which are conducive to good health and longevity (Whalley and Deary 2001). Highly intelligent people can not only process cognitive information rapidly but are also often capable of remaining physiologically fit, with well-functioning nervous systems. In contrast, an examination of individuals with significant cognitive deficits or cognitive impairments suggests an association between low-functioning brains and higher mortality risk. For example, death rates for individuals with learning disabilities are often found to be higher than those found in the general population (McGuigan et al. 1995).

Furthermore, individuals of lower intelligence may have experienced insults to their brains from disease or from external trauma (Friedman 1994). Thus, it appears that individuals at the extremes in intellectual functioning (very high or very low IQs) may experience very different life trajectories. Note, however, that these predictions from brain biology go against the stereotype of the brainy weakling. In other words, it is not clear from this biological analysis how to reconcile what the popular wisdom tells us about brains versus brawn.

Might the Terman participants have been able to resist disease and suffer fewer brain insults throughout their lives? Findings from the Nun Study (Snowdon 1997) point to the importance of "exercising" and developing cognitive abilities in order to continue to function (both cognitively and physically) later in life. The Nun Study suggests that advanced cognitive functioning may modify the clinical expression of disease and help avert some of the physical decline associated with aging (Snowdon 1997; Snowdon et al. 1996). Cognitive functioning has been shown to predict longevity even when other important factors, including age, gender, and education, are controlled for (Smits et al. 1999). Thus, might the high intellectual capacity of the Terman cohort and their potential for complex cognitive functions have protected them from morbidity and risk of premature mortality as they aged?

Although biological factors have thus been proposed as linking intelligence and longevity, few data are available to suggest a robust relationship between intelligence and longevity. Very smart people die at high rates in their 60s and 70s, just as do less intelligent people. This is probably because many other health-relevant factors enter the picture during one's lifetime. By using a longitudinal data set containing information about highly intelligent individuals' health and longevity, we can gain some understanding of the effects of elevated intelligence. What are the possible psychosocial and lifestyle factors that become relevant?

The Terman Participants' Longevity

Because Terman only admitted promising, highly intelligent children into his study, it is probable that all of the Terman participants were biologically positioned to maintain their health. Further, because of their access to schooling and health care, we might expect that this sample would live much longer than the general population.

The Terman participants' mortality rates are compared to the United States 1910 cohort mortality rates in Figure 1. (The Terman participants were, on average, born in 1910.) Some of the numbers presented are estimates, due to incomplete population data.

When the Terman participants' mortality rates are compared to the mortality rates of the general U.S. population born in 1910, a major observation emerges. Intelligent people in Terman's sample lived longer than their general population peers, even after taking into account the fact (artifact) that all the Terman participants, by study design, lived at least until age 10; *however,* the patterns of mortality risk and overall risk later in life are *not* strikingly different (see Fig. 1). The patterns are similar.

Furthermore, in hazard regression analyses, intelligence is not related to participants' longevity *within* the Terman sample. This finding holds for both men and women in this sample. Although this null result is likely due to the restricted range of intelligence scores among the Terman participants, it is con-

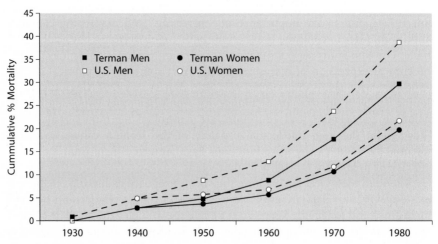

Fig. 1. Comparing Terman life cycle cumulative mortality rates with 1910 cohort life tables. Figure copyright Howard S. Friedman. Reprinted by permission

sistent with the more general finding. Variations in IQ at the extreme (i.e., above 135) do not predict longevity, just as being in the Terman sample does not predict a markedly long life. A direct, biological relationship between intelligence and longevity may be overwhelmed by other variables that may more directly impact an individual's life path.

Health Behavior Influences on Paths to Longevity

If the biological health of the organism is not enough to explain mortality risk, might key health behaviors be critical? Highly intelligent individuals are certainly better able to receive and understand health information, and so seem more likely to utilize health-relevant information than someone who doesn't understand the message. This ability is relevant both to the avoidance of harmful substances (e.g., tobacco products) and the utilization of beneficial substances (e.g., medication). Further, high intelligence might lead to better decision making in regards to health behaviors.

Health-related behaviors, especially tobacco and alcohol abuse, are commonly targeted today in interventions designed to prevent disease and increase longevity, but earlier in the 20th century, messages were mixed. Nevertheless, although the dangers of tobacco and alcohol were not as well documented as they are today, it was clear by the 1950s (when the Terman participants were in their 40s) that heavy drinking and smoking were not the royal road to health.

Among the Terman participants, alcohol consumption was well assessed in 1950 and 1960. Smoking was assessed retrospectively in 1991–1992 and is biased in that direct information is not available on those who smoked heavily and died young. In the total Terman sample 20 % never or rarely drank, 54 % reported being moderate drinkers, and 27 % reported being heavy drinkers (Men: 15 % never or rarely, 51 % moderate, 35 % heavy. Women: 26 % never or rarely, 57 % moderate, 17 % heavy). Among Terman men, alcohol consumption is not significantly related to intelligence ($r(691) = 0.03$, $p > .05$). Among Terman women, alcohol consumption is inversely related to intelligence ($r(537) = -0.11$, $p < .05$).

Data from a nationally representative sample study conducted in the mid-1960s (Calahan et al. 1969) suggest that among men who are comparable in age to the Terman participants, 44 % of men rarely or never drank, 34 % were moderate drinkers, and 22 % were heavy drinkers. Among women, 64 % rarely or never drank, 35 % were moderate drinkers, and 1 % were heavy drinkers. These data suggest that the Terman participants were heavier drinkers than the U.S. population average.

Thirty-nine percent of the total sample of Terman participants were non-smokers, 21 % smoked 1–320 cigarettes a year,[1] 20 % smoked 321–880 cigarettes

---

[1] Cigarettes smoked per year was computed by multiplying the total number of years the participant reported smoking by the average number of cigarettes per day smoked during those years.

a year, and 21 % smoked 881–3600 cigarettes per year. U.S. population statistics suggest that, in 1965 (the first year that smoking rates were fully documented by the National Center for Health Statistics), 42 % of white adults were smokers (Epidemiology and Statistics Unit 1999). Although detailed statistics for 1965 are not available, this information suggests that the percent of the Terman sample that smoked in adulthood (61 %) exceeded population norms.

These health-related behaviors are related to premature mortality in the Terman sample. Specifically, alcohol consumption and smoking are inversely related to longevity, with heavy drinkers (relative hazard = 1.25 for men and 1.23 for women) and smokers (relative hazard = 1.19 for men and 1.41 for women) dying significantly earlier than their peers who did not engage in consumptive behaviors (Friedman et al. 1995). Although all the Terman participants were extremely intelligent, they were not protected from a fate similar to their less intelligent counterparts who engaged in health-compromising behaviors.

Psychological Influences on Paths to Longevity

A variety of research suggests that individuals' psychological health and adaptation play an active role in determining their health and longevity (Friedman 1991/2000 a). In addition to the health behavior mechanisms, psychological health status and personality traits are important to understanding intelligence and health, as individuals find themselves in different situations along life's pathways.

The link between mental and physical health has long been speculated about, and research of the past decade documents the associations among psychological health, cognitive health, and physical health. For example, stress and anxiety are closely tied to psychological strength, cognitive abilities / cognitive coping, and health problems (Anda et al. 1993, Brummett et al. 1998; Jonas and Mussolino 2000; Kamarack and Jennings 1991). However, the relations among these constructs is often complex. For example, among the elderly, depression has been discussed as a risk factor for cognitive decline, which in turn has been discussed as a risk factor for mortality (Geerlings et al. 2000). The reverse has also been documented; psychological health has been shown to facilitate cognitive functioning among the elderly (Poon et al. 1992). Further, illness can bring on depression and cognitive decline.

Among the Terman participants, psychological health is not significantly correlated with intelligence. However, our findings suggest that psychological adjustment is positively related to longevity in the Terman sample (Martin et al. 1995). In 1950, the "Termites" were asked about tendencies toward nervousness, anxiety, or nervous breakdown. In addition, personal conferences with participants and with their family members provided information about the Terman sample's mental health status. Based on this and on previous related information in the files dating back a decade, Terman's team then categorized each on a three-point scale of mental difficulty: satisfactory adjustment, some maladjustment, or serious maladjustment. Survival analyses show that for males, mental difficulty as of 1950 significantly predicted mortality risk through 1991, in the expected direction (relative hazard = 1.30, $p < 0.01$ for males; rh = 1.12, ns., for females). Similar results were found on a measure we constructed of poor psychological adjustment as self-reported in 1950 (significant mortality risk for males, $p < 0.05$, but not for females).

Although personality has been defined in many ways, most commonly personality is conceptualized as "the dynamic organization within an individual that determines his characteristic behavior and thought" (Allport 1961, p. 28). Most importantly here, this habitual pattern of perceiving, thinking, and behaving leads some individuals to gravitate toward healthy environments, whereas others tend to habitually place themselves in threatening situations (Caspi and Bem 1990; Friedman 1991/2000 a, b). These movements of individuals towards more or less suitable situations are both a product of and an influence on personality (McCrae and Costa 1995; Friedman 2000 b).

Some of the most remarkable findings from the Terman cohort suggest the importance of childhood personality in influencing the risk of premature mortality. The individuals' way of relating to their environment appears to be extremely important in determining their life paths. Specifically, parents' and teachers' assessments of the Terman participants' personality traits have been examined. Conscientiousness, lack of cheerfulness, and permanency of mood (males only) are related to increased longevity among this highly intelligent group (Friedman et al. 1993; Friedman et al. 1995 a; Schwartz et al. 1995). In particular, childhood conscientiousness appears to have wide-ranging effects on health, affecting longevity in diverse ways (Friedman et al. 1995 a). Additionally, personality qualities are thought to influence individuals' tendencies to participate in health-promoting and health-compromising behaviors and stress-management capabilities beginning in childhood and continuing through adulthood (Block et al. 1988; John et al. 1994; Markey et al. 2002).

Social Influences on Paths to Longevity

The effects of social support, life transitions, and stressful events on health and longevity are all well documented, even if the mechanisms are not always fully understood (Friedman 2002). For the most part, the social milieu that surrounded the Terman children consisted of white, middle class environments capable of providing opportunities for health and success. This positive context, combined with the Terman participants' intellectual capacity, placed them at an advantage (Whalley and Deary 2001). However, although these factors may have served to eliminate some of life's challenges, many of life's stressors remained. Stressful life events can trigger chronic autonomic arousal, and this continuous arousal can cause lasting changes in basic psychological and intellectual processes, as well as in health behaviors.

The Terman data provide an opportunity to evaluate how stressful social experiences influence pathways to longevity. In particular, we have looked at the children whose parents either did or did not divorce before the child reached age 21 (Friedman et al. 1995 b; Tucker et al. 1996, 1997). Parental divorce is an important social event to evaluate because it epitomizes what a stress-producing event is; it leads to a reduction in social support, a drastic period of transition, and the experience of an uncontrollable situation.

Among the Terman participants, children of divorced parents faced a one-third greater mortality risk than people whose parents remained married until the children reached age 21. Although a minority (13 %) of the Terman cohort experienced parental divorce, a majority of children may face parental divorce in contemporary society; so these long-term health implications of this stressful social experience need to be considered. Interestingly, within the Terman sample, parental divorce and personality traits appear to be independent predictors of longevity. However, when considered in combination, the trait of childhood conscientiousness and the experience of parental divorce is equal to the effect of gender on longevity, which is one of the most robust predictors of longevity (see Fig. 2).

In the Terman cohort, the experience of parental divorce is also associated with experiencing the breakup of one's own marriage. Individuals who report having their parents' divorce also report more stressful childhoods and are more likely to have less stable relationships as adults. This relationship instability appears to influence individuals' psychological and physical health, making

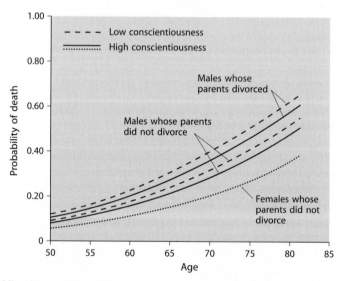

Fig. 2. Childhood personality, childhood stress, and longevity in the Terman sample. Note: the probability of dying by age seventy is greater than 0.40 (more than 40 %) for high-risk males, less than 0.30 for low risk males, and only about 0.20 for low risk females. Figure copyright Howard S. Friedman and Joseph Schwartz. Reprinted by permission.

them vulnerable to disease and reduced longevity (Tucker et al. 1999). Social influences thus take their place beside behavioral and psychological influences in longevity in this intelligent group.

Conclusions

The Terman data set provides researchers with a rich opportunity to explore the paths to longevity among a highly intelligent cohort of individuals who were successful in elementary school in 1922. Although the Terman participants were highly intelligent, they often behaved in ways and experienced various psychosocial issues throughout their lives that impaired their health, leading to mortality risks that, in many cases, were not strikingly different than those experienced by a much less intelligent population. It appears that once an individual reaches a certain, average level of intelligence, other aspects of the individual become more important in determining health status and longevity. Intelligence does not directly predict longevity in this sample, a sample of restricted range in IQ.

Rather, among the Terman participants, health-related behaviors (substance use), psychological adjustment, personality traits, and social relationships all predict longevity. Individuals who are conscientious, well-adjusted and in stable families and who minimize their smoking and drinking live longer. What is somewhat counterintuitive and previously not well understood is the empirical support derived from analyses with the Terman data suggesting that even highly intelligent people, just like their peers of average intelligence, are highly susceptible to behavioral and psychosocial threats to health and longevity. While high intelligence is advantageous in certain domains, it is not decisively advantageous when considering health and longevity.

Why would many of these intelligent people drink and smoke heavily and be often unable to straighten out their psychological and social lives? Perhaps we or they overestimate their wisdom. As the African proverb asserts, "A wise man never knows all; only fools know everything." Or, perhaps they recognized their limits, but intelligence does not necessarily lead to self-control. As Shakespeare put it, "The fool doth think he is wise, but the wise man knows himself to be a fool" (As You Like It). Or perhaps these highly intelligent and privileged men and women simply outsmarted themselves, seeking fashionable or exciting lives. As Philippe Quinault said, "It is not wise to be wiser than necessary." [Ce n'est pas etre sage, Qu'etre sage plus qu'il faut." (Armide)].

Intelligent individuals are often stereotyped as mentally strong yet physically weak and nerdy. Almost a century ago, Lewis Terman sought to overturn this stereotype by instigating a vast longitudinal investigation of highly intelligent individuals. What the data have shown us is that while smart people are not weak and nerdy, and do have certain advantages in maintaining their health, they are not invincible to behavioral and psychosocial influences that interact with biology to determine mortality risk. The Terman data and related findings continue to point to the importance of understanding the multifaceted nature of health.

Acknowledgements

This research is supported by grant AG 08825 of the National Institute on Aging. The opinions are those of the authors and not necessarily of the NIA.

References

Anda R, Williamson D, Jones D, Marcera C, Eaker E, Glassman A, Marks J (1993) Depressed affect, hopelessness, and the risk of ischemic heart disease in a cohort of U.S. Adults. Epidemiology 4: 285–294

Allport G (1961) Pattern and growth in personality. Holt, Rinehart, & Winston, New York

Block J, Block JH, Keyes S (1988) Longitudinally foretelling drug usage in adolescence: Early childhood personality and environmental precursors. Child Devel 59: 336–355

Brummett BH, Babyak MA, Barefoot JC, Bosworth HB, Clapp-Channing NE, Siegler MIC, Williams RB, Mark DB (1998) Social support and hostility as predictors of depressive symptoms in cardiac patients one month after hospitalization: A prospective study. Psychosomatic Med 60: 707–713

Calahan D, Cisis IH, Crossley HM (1969) American drinking practices: a national study of drinking behavior and attitudes. Monograph of the Rutgers Center of Alcohol Studies No. 6. New Brunswick, NJ, Rutgers Center of Alcohol Studies

Caspi A, Bem DJ (1990) Personality continuity and change across the life course. In: Pervin LA (ed) Handbook of personality: Theory and research. The Guilford Press, New York, pp. 549–575

Epidemiology and Statistics Unit (1999) Trends in cigarette smoking. [On-Line] http: www.lungusa.org/data/smoke/smoke-1.pdf

Friedman HS (1991/2000 a) Self-Healing Personality: Why Some People Achieve Health and Others Succumb to Illness. Re-published by: (www.iuniverse.com), New York

Friedman HS (1994) Intelligence and health. In: Sternberg RJ (ed) Encyclopedia of intelligence. MacMillan, New York, pp. 521–525

Friedman HS (2000 b) Long-term relations of personality and health: Dynamisms, mechanisms, tropisms. J Pers 68: 1089–1108

Friedman HS (2002) Health psychology. Second edition. Upper Saddle River, NJ, Prentice Hall

Friedman HS, Tucker JS, Tomlinson-Keasey C, Schwartz J, Wingard DL, Criqui MH (1993) Does childhood personality predict longevity? J Pers Soc Psychol 65: 176–185

Friedman HS, Tucker JS, Schwartz J, Martin LR, Tomlinson-Keasey C, Wingard DL, Criqui MH (1995 a) Childhood conscientiousness and longevity: Health behaviors and cause of death. J Pers Soc Psychol 68: 696–703

Friedman HS, Tucker JS, Schwartz JE, Tomlinson-Keasey C, Martin LR, Wingard DL, Criqui M (1995 b) Psychosocial and behavioral predictors of longevity: The aging and death of the "Termites." Am Psychol 50: 69–78

Geerlings MI, Schoevers RA, Beekman AT, Jonker C, Deeg DJ, Schman AHJ, Bouter LM, Van Tilburg W (2000) Depression and risk of cognitive and Alzheimer's disease. Results of two prospective community-based studies in the Netherlands. Brit J Psychiat 176: 568–575

John OP, Caspi A, Moffitt TE, Stouthamer-Loeber M (1994) The "Little Five": Exploring the nomological network of the Five-Factor Model of personality in adolescent boys. Child Devel 65: 160–178

Jonas BS, Mussolino ME (2000) Symptoms of depression as a prospective risk factor for stroke. Psychosomatic Med 62: 463–471

Kamarack TW, Jennings JR (1991) Biobehavioral factors in sudden cardiac death. Psychol Bull 109: 42–75

Markey CN, Ericksen AJ, Markey PM, Tinsley BJ (2002) Personality and family determinants of preadolescents' participation in health-compromising and health-promoting behaviors. Adolesc Family Health, in press

Martin LR, Friedman HS, Tucker JS, Schwartz JE, Criqui MH, Wingard DL, Tomlinson-Keasey C (1995) An archival prospective study of mental health and longevity. Health Psychol 14: 381–387

McCrae RR, Costa PT (1995) Trait explanations in personality psychology. Eur J Pers 9: 231–252

McGuigan SM, Hollins S, Attard M (1995) Age-specific standardized mortality rates in people with learning disability. J Intel Disabil Res 39: 527–531

Poon LW, Messner S, Martin P, Noble (1992) The influences of cognitive resources on adaptation and age. Int J Aging Human Devel 34: 31–36

Schwartz JE, Friedman HS, Tucker JS, Tomlinson-Keasey C, Wingard DL, Criqui MH (1995) Sociodemographic and psychosocial factors in childhood as predictors of adult mortality. Am J Publ Health 85: 1237–1245

Smits CH, Deeg DJ, Kriegsman DM, Schmand B (1999) Cognitive functioning and health as determinants of mortality in an older population. Am J Epidemiol 150: 978–986

Snowden DA (1997) Aging and Alzheimer's disease: Lessons from the Nun Study. Gerontology 37: 150–156

Snowden DA, Kemper SJ, Mortimer JA, Greiner LH, Wekstein DR, Markesbery WR (1996) Linguistic ability early in life and cognitive function and Alzheimer's disease in late life: Findings from the Nun Study. JAMA 275: 528–532

Terman LM (1925) Genetic studies of genius: Mental and physical traits of a thousand gifted children. Stanford University Press, Stanford, CA

Terman LM, Oden MH (1947) Genetic studies of genius, IV. The gifted children grown up: Twenty-five years follow-up of a superior group. Stanford University Press, Stanford, CA

Tucker JS, Friedman HS, Wingard DL, Schwartz JE (1996) Marital history at midlife as a predictor of longevity: Alternative explanations to the protective effect of marriage. Health Psychol 15: 94–101

Tucker JS, Friedman HS, Schwartz JE, Criqui MH, Tomlinson-Keasey C, Wingard D, Martin LR (1997) Parental divorce: Effects on individual behavior longevity. J Pers Soc Psychol 73: 381–391

Tucker JS, Schwartz JE, Clark KM, Friedman HS (1999) Age-related changes in the association of social network ties with mortality risk. Psychol Aging 14: 564–571

Whalley LJ, Deary IJ (2001) Longitudinal cohort study of childhood IQ and survival up to age 76. Brit Med J 322: 819–829

Subject Index

Printing: Mercedes-Druck, Berlin
Binding: Stein+Lehmann, Berlin